Dr. Ridgway is the author of *How to Treat Your Dogs and Cats with Over-the-Counter Drugs, How to Treat Your Dogs and Cats with Over-the-Counter Drugs Companion Edition*, eighteen professional journal articles, and five professional auto-tutorials.

THE TRUTH about DOG and CAT TREATMENTS AND ANOMALIES

ROBERT L. RIDGWAY, DVM

iUniverse LLC
Bloomington

The Truth about Dog and Cat Treatments and Anomalies

iUniverse books may be ordered through booksellers or by contacting:

iUniverse
1663 Liberty Drive
Bloomington, IN 47403
www.iuniverse.com
1-800-Authors (1-800-288-4677)

ISBN: 978-1-4759-9673-9 (sc)
ISBN: 978-1-4759-9674-6 (hc)
ISBN: 978-1-4759-9675-3 (e)

Library of Congress Control Number: 2013911736

Printed in the United States of America.

iUniverse rev. date: 10/28/2013

To the College of Veterinary Medicine, Kansas State University, and the College of Veterinary Medicine, University of California–Davis

Dr. Paul McRae, DVM, and Dr. Bob Playter, DVM

CONTENTS

LIST OF TABLES

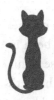 # FOREWORD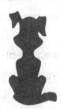

If you have had a dog or cat for any period of time, you have probably seen a worrisome condition, such as vomiting, cough, limping, or diarrhea, and wondered what to do. This fine book is a good place to start making decisions about whether to give an over-the-counter medication to your pet or to take it to the veterinarian. The book clearly describes more than 150 problems you might encounter. The book describes these conditions and guides readers about what medications and dosages would be appropriate and how long to continue treatment. More importantly, the book explains when conditions need to be evaluated by a veterinarian. Additionally, the book advises the reader about how to prevent these conditions from occurring in the first place.

Dr. Ridgway is a well-known veterinarian. He has written many scientific articles as well as several books. He is an expert in his field. Having this book by your side is like having your own expert by your side to guide you! Dr. Ridgway writes in an easy-to-understand way that is devoid of medical terminology. This makes the book even more valuable and easy to understand.

I would like to tell you something about the author. After receiving his doctorate degree in veterinary medicine from Kansas State University, Dr. Ridgway completed a residency at the University of California. He is board certified by the American College of Preventive Medicine and the American College of Laboratory Animal Medicine. Dr. Ridgway spent his early career years in the United States

Army. He traveled frequently to Germany to select dogs for all of the military branches. To train such dogs is very expensive and starts with selecting the best dogs available. Obviously, this was a difficult job that only a real expert could do. A lot of government money rested on his decision!

Dr. Ridgway retired from the army as a lieutenant colonel and went into private practice in Orlando, Florida. He has been in veterinary medicine for more than forty years. In the course of his practice, Dr. Ridgway saw a real need for some way to guide his pet's owners about what to do when their pets seemed to have problems. Some people brought their pets in for conditions that could have been treated at home. Worse yet, some people delayed seeking professional help when it was actually a serious emergency. To me, this book is a fine guide to differentiate between such conditions. It will save the lives of many pets and will save owners lots of money.

Note, however, that Dr. Ridgway's book is not meant to replace regular visits to your veterinarian. In fact, Dr. Ridgway strongly advocates such visits as well as a program of preventive medicine to keep pets healthy. Furthermore, one of the great values of this book is its encouragement for the reader to recognize when a visit to the veterinarian is needed and to not avoid delays in such visits, which could cause professional help to become much more prolonged and expensive.

For all the above reasons, I will keep this book close at hand. I am thrilled to add this book to my reference library and will refer to it often. My dog and my cat will surely benefit from Dr. Ridgway's expertise—and so will you.

Charles H. Beckmann, MD, FACP, FACC, FAHA
Professor of Medicine, Retired
Uniformed Services University of the Health Sciences
Bethesda, Maryland, and San Antonio, Texas

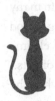# PREFACE

You will find that this book is written in common, everyday language to help nonveterinarians understand the content. If I told you to look at the *medial canthus*, you might not understand me. However, if I say, "Look at the corner of the eye next to the nose," you will understand.

In this book there are more than 152 anomalies and/or remedies. By following the simple instructions, any person can treat his or her pets at home for a variety conditions.

In any situation, the best solution is to have the pet see a qualified veterinarian. However, there are conditions that prevent folks from doing so. Finances and distance from clinics are at the top of the list, and other reasons may come to mind.

The format of this book is to describe a condition and, if possible, a treatment plan, followed by suggestions for preventing the condition from occurring. Not all subjects have a treatment or preventive suggestion; some treatments are best left to a veterinarian, and some conditions cannot be prevented.

Remember that there is a limit to what can be done for pets with over-the-counter drugs. I have selected the subjects I discuss for two reasons. The conditions are either common or frequently seen in a day-to-day veterinary practice, or the subjects give owners a broad resource written in everyday language. This book does not cover every ailment that may affect a pet. I was not trying to produce the best-looking doorstop you could find.

I may suggest an over-the-counter drug treatment, or I may

suggest taking a pet to see a veterinarian. Why refer to a veterinarian? There are conditions that need prescription drugs, blood work, x-rays, surgery, and other procedures.

After the treatment discussions, I sometimes offer prevention suggestions that may allow the owner to avoid the condition. In many cases, however, there is not much an owner can do. Maintaining a good preventive medicine program allows early detection of unwelcome health conditions, which can save money and extend the life of pets.

I'm often asked if it is necessary to go to the veterinarian when the pet seems to be doing fine. My answer is that my physician sees me routinely every six months. There have been times when he has picked up issues early, preventing further development of a potentially serious condition. A wellness program is a heck of a lot cheaper than treating a full-blown medical issue. My answer to the question is always yes; following a regular wellness program, regardless of your pet's apparent health, is the best thing you can do for your pet buddy.

I have provided many charts that allow you to look up a pet's weight and give the correct medication dosage for that weight. This eliminates the need to manually calculate dosages. However, you— and you alone—make the decision to treat your pet with over-the-counter drugs. This book is only a guide, and the dosages provided are safe for most pets *if you follow the recommendations*. There is always a chance a pet may be allergic to a drug. This cannot be known until it happens. If an adverse reaction does occur, you will need to see the pet's doctor immediately. Never repeat the medicine that caused the reaction in your pet.

The authors and publisher specifically disclaim any and all liability arising directly or indirectly from the use or application of any information contained in this publication.

Pets often become a part of the family. They are our buddies, and we want the best for them. The best option for the treatment of your pet is the pet's doctor. Veterinarians have been extensively trained in the art of medicine dedicated to the treatment of animals. A veterinarian is always the best approach for medical information and treatment.

When using any drug, it is important that the proper diagnosis is made first. Understanding the condition that you intend to treat is essential. The next step is to decide on the best medication for that condition. After the selection of medication, the proper amount of the drug must be decided. This requires your full attention to prevent you from overdosing your pet.

Drug dosages are based on weight—a given amount of drug per pound or per kilogram that the pet weighs. It normally takes a bit of math to calculate the proper dosage. In this book, that step has been done for you. All you need know for a proper dosage of a drug is the weight of your pet.

Know your pet's weight. Use the dosage chart and look up the dosage according to that weight. Administer the drug in the recommended dosage only. Do not believe or think that if a little bit of drug is good, then a lot more should be better. This kind of thinking kills pets.

CHAPTER 1

SKIN DISORDERS

Now this is not the end. It is not even the beginning of the
end. But it is, perhaps, the end of the beginning.
—Sir Winston Churchill

The skin is the largest organ of the body. Skin may account for 12–24 percent of a pet's body weight. The skin has many functions, which include being an enclosure barrier, regulating temperature, producing pigment, producing vitamin D, functioning as a sensor organ, growing hair, and stretching and shrinking. The skin organ can be easily damaged, but it has an uncanny ability to repair and mend itself from many different kinds of trauma. At times, the skin needs help healing, and you need to provide this help to allow your pet's skin to repair.

I recently repaired a severe burn on the back of a small breed of dog that will look like new without a visible scar due to the unique reparability of the skin. This organ has hair that gives color to the pet. Unfortunately, a lack of attention to our pet's skin issues can result in major dermatologic problems. In this chapter, we will address many skin issues as well as others that normally can be prevented with simple attentiveness to such things as crustiness, scaling, nodules, hair loss, nonhealing wounds, excessive scratching at the skin, and other problems that can occur to the largest organ of the body.

1

YOUR PET, YOUR CHILDREN, YOU, AND MRSA

What the heck is MRSA? Methicillin-Resistant Staphylococcus Aureus (MRSA) is often called by its acronym and is pronounced "murr-sir" for short or just called staph. Methicillin is a penicillin salt used to treat bacterial infections. Staphylococci can also be found on the skin, in skin glands, in the nasal passages—and other mucous membranes of warm-blooded animals—and in a variety of food products.

MRSA is most commonly found in the nose or nasal passages and around the anus of dogs and cats. However, it can be found in other areas too. I read about a cat that had MRSA on its toes, up its neck, and into its ears. Staphylococci can cause infections of tissue cells of the gums, heart, lungs, bones, and in wounds and open sores. Just about any part of the body can become infected by this and many other organisms.

The problem is not just MRSA; organisms such as *Streptococci pseudintermedius* (MRSP) can become resistant to bacteria. Pets commonly carry MRSP or streptococcus infections, and humans tend to carry MRSA. Streptococcus infections tend to be found in open wounds and recent surgery sites as well as the nose and around the anus. Resistance is most often caused by prolonged use of antibiotics working on fast-developing bacteria that sets the stage for bacterial resistance. All animals have bacteria on their bodies; most of the time, this bacteria is in check between the different species that live on the body. Bacteria are one-celled organisms that can reproduce rapidly and develop resistance from mutations that occur quickly.

If your pet/pets have any antibiotic-resistant bug, is it a risk to your children and to you? Most would say that getting a resistant bug from a pet is very uncommon, but it can, does, and has happened. If you have a bacterial-resistant bacterium on your pet, you should seek the advice of your family physician and let your physician help you with this problem as it relates to your children and you. Certainly if any family member obtains an infection of any kind and you know that your pet/pets have a drug-resistant infection, you need to make your family physician aware of the situation. This information will help your physician. The young are more apt to obtain an infection from a bacteria-resistant pet since they play with the pet and may be kissing the pet or touching areas where they should not touch, such as the nose or the anal areas of pets. Many people kiss their pets, and any pet with a bacterial-resistant infection should not be kissed until it has healed.

TREATMENT
This type of infection should be under the direct guidance and treatment plan of your pet's veterinarian. It has the potential to be dangerous to family members. However, it is thought that transmission from pets to people is rare. If the rare infection happens to be one of your family members, it could be serious—and possibly fatal.

PREVENTION
The best way to prevent this condition is to have a good wellness plan and have health checks at least two times per year. If disease conditions are noted at these checkups—and if diseases are present or caught in early stages—further development can often be prevented. This saves big bucks in the long run since a healthy pet is cheaper than one being treated for any health condition.

PET GROOMING

Many cats and dogs with long hair are not groomed properly and have mats on the body that allow for skin infections, flea infestations, and dirt and grime accumulations. The issue of grooming is a day-to-day commitment for the pet owner. Merely brushing the pet daily will keep the mats away. However, unlike an apple a day will keep the doctor away, it is not so when it comes to pet grooming. My personal experience with brushing a cat is that the cat loves it and purrs all the time it is being brushed. The cat actually shows up on time to be groomed every evening about shower time.

There is an instrument called a FURminator that is an excellent tool for ridding the pet of dead hairs in the body coat. The FURminator can be purchased online or at pet stores. By using the FURminator, many dead hairs are removed. With the use of the FURminator, you ensure that there will never be hair mats on your pet. You have to use the FURminator. You cannot purchase it and let it sit on a shelf and expect the pet not to have hair mats.

The coat of any furry animal has three types of hair: anagen (new hairs), catagen (middle-age hairs or between the anagen and telogen hairs), and telogen (resting or dead hairs). The telogen hairs are often left on tables and chairs when a pet gets nervous or scared. Telogen hairs are released due to the so-called *erector pili* muscles contracting when the pet is excited or frightened.

PREVENTION

Grooming prevents clumping of hair and prevents lameness due to foot issues caused by matted hair on the feet and between the toes. It prevents dirt and grime accumulation under hair mats, which often result in skin infections. Prevent skin infections by grooming your pet, which shows your pride in the pet—and the pet looks so much better.

HAIR LOSS OR MATTING ON THE
TAIL OF CATS AND DOGS

Many cats and dogs will start to lose the hair on the top side of the tail or so-called dorsal side of the tail. Normally this syndrome starts with a small area of hair loss in dogs; in cats, the hair on the tail starts to become matted, and there is an accumulation of waxy, oily accumulation of the tail hair. This is due to the oil secretion from the so-called sebaceous glands that are concentrated on the top or dorsal side of the tail.

This syndrome is common in dogs. It often starts with a small area of hair loss that gets larger with time. A small area of hair loss is often the first sign in dogs. Normally the lesion is about 2.5–5 cm [1–2 inches] below the tail head. The hair loss area may be scaly, greasy, and have an increased darkening of the skin.

It is not uncommon for dogs to have a secondary infection associated with the hair loss. This, however, is not a 100 percent occurring sign. If a secondary infection does occur, you will need to see your pet's favorite doctor for antibiotics.

In cats, the oily secretions cause a stripe of matted hair with a waxy, oily accumulation. As with the dog, the cat's tail may become darker in the affected area. In both the dog and the cat, the discoloration tends to be black or at least dark. In the cat, the lesion is normally confined to the tail, and there is no other skin involved. This is not necessarily so in the dog; many dogs have seborrhea secretions on other areas of the body.

Stud tail is a cosmetic disease and does not affect the quality of life of the pet; normally the prognosis is good for this syndrome. Fortunately, it is uncommon in cats. However, this syndrome is rather common in dogs of all sizes.

TREATMENT

The treatment of choice for cats and dogs is castration or surgical neutering. In the dog, castration may induce partial to complete lesion regression or prevent any further development of the syndrome. Improvement is seen within two months.

Surgery is not an instant fix like a lot of people like to think in this modern world. In cats, surgery may not resolve the issue, but it may help prevent further development of the problem. Surgical excision of the lesion has been tried, but it is not very effective since the lesion may reoccur within four years. This option is not feasible due to needing to repeat the surgery.

This is a personal decision you will have to make if faced with this issue. In cats, regular grooming of the matted hair and combing may be necessary, especially for cats that are poor groomers. I would recommend the FURminator for helping to keep the tail hair groomed. The FURminator is somewhat expensive, but I have found it to be very easy to use and very effective. I know of no other grooming tool that works as well.

Omega-3 fatty acids have been of some benefit; depending on the animal's size, doses can range from 500 mg to 3000 mg. I suggest about

180 mg EPA of omega-3 fatty acids per ten pounds of body weight. You be the judge about the effectiveness by trying a dose of fish oil (omega-3 fatty acids), but remember that no treatment is instant. It takes time to be effective. Seborrhea shampoos used every two to seven days have been used with some success since they cut the oily accumulations and may improve smell. See Table 1.1.

The dose to be given is determined by the weight of the pet. You can also purchase fish oil. Dump the oil into a small container—and give the same dose according to the following charts. Dealing with fish oil capsules is anything but convenient. It is a messy way to obtain the omega-3 acids, and Nordic Naturals can be purchased at vitamin shops and online. Type "Nordic Naturals" in the search line, and the site to order online pops up. The products come with a calculated dose dropper that is easy to use. The website is www.omega-direct.com. Click on products, and then click on pet products, or you can make a free call 1-800-595-2714.

PREVENTION

This is a so-called idiopathic condition, which means that we do not know what triggers the condition. There is really not much you can do to prevent it. If it is going to happen, it will occur. You will at least know what it is and what can be done if you elect to do so. If you have a wellness plan, it will normally be diagnosed early. This will prevent further development in your pet of the so-called stud tail.

A problem with capsules is that more oil gets on one's hands than into the pet. You could cut the capsules, pour the oil in a container, and then dose the oil from the container at the same dosage as Nordic Naturals from Table 1.1. Nordic Naturals has worked out the dosing and has an easy way of getting the correct dose without any fuss.

Table 1.1 *Omega-3 Fatty Acids*

Doses for omega 3-fatty acids are
courtesy of Nordic Naturals.
Suggested daily dose for dogs
one teaspoon = 5 ml (4600 mg)

Weight	Serving	Servings per Bottle	EPA	DHA	Total Omega-3s
2–4 lbs. (.9–1.8 kg)	0.25 cc or ml	240	35 mg	21 mg	71 mg
5–9 lbs. (2.2–4.0 kg)	1.0 cc or ml	60	138 mg	83 mg	285 mg
10–19 lbs. (4.5–8.6 kg)	2.0 cc or ml	30	276 mg	166 mg	570 mg
20–39 lbs. (9–17.6 kg)	0.5 teaspoon (2.5 cc or ml)	189	345 mg	207 mg	713 mg
40–59 lbs. (18–26.7 kg)	1.0 teaspoon (5.0 cc or ml)	94	690 mg	414 mg	1426 mg
60–79 lbs. (27.2–35.8 kg)	1.5 teaspoons (7.5 cc or ml)	63	1035 mg	621 mg	2139 mg
80–99 lbs. (36.2–44.9 kg)	2.0 teaspoons (10 cc or ml)	47	1380 mg	828 mg	2952 mg
100 lbs. (45.35 kg)	3.0 teaspoons (15 ml)	31	2070 mg	1242 mg	4278 mg

lbs. = pounds, kg = kilograms, cc = ml or ml = cc

Suggested daily dose for dogs
Use of soft gel capsules, for every 20 pounds (9.0 kg) of body weight

Weight	Serving	EPA	DHA	Total Omega-3s
20 lbs.	1 soft gel	150 mg	90 mg	310 mg

Suggested daily dose for cats
one teaspoon = 5 ml (4600 mg)

Weight	Serving	Servings per Bottle	EPA	DHA	Total Omega-3s
2–4 lbs. (.90–1.8 kg)	0.25 cc or ml	249	35 mg	21 mg	71 mg
5–9 lbs. (2.26–4.0 kg)	0.5 cc or ml	120	69 mg	41 mg	143 mg
10–14 lbs. (4.53–6.35)	0.75 cc or ml	80	104 mg	62 mg	214 mg
15–20 lbs. (6.8–9.0 kg)	1.0 cc or ml	60	138 mg	83 mg	285 mg
Over 20 lbs. (9.0 kg)	1.25 cc or ml	48	173 mg	104 mg	356 mg

lbs. = pounds, kg = kilograms, cc = ml or ml = cc

DOG AND CAT BLEEDING SKIN

The most obvious sign of bleeding in a dog or cat is the presence of blood on the surface of the pet. The very first thing one must do is not to lose one's cool. Stay calm if you feel yourself becoming excited or apprehensive. Count to ten and take a deep breath. Once you have settled down, your next step is to determine how much trauma is present, where the trauma is, and if it is something you can treat—or if it is a job for the pet's doctor.

To determine if you need to take the pet to see the doctor, think about open wounds on yourself. If a wound on your body is not bad, you tend to treat it yourself; if it is bad, you go to your physician. Use the same evaluation system for your pet as you would for yourself.

You can treat bleeding wounds effectively with *Quick Clot* or *Pet Clot*. This is an amazing, relatively new product on the market that works for people, small pets, and large pets. It stops bleeding very quickly.

TREATMENT

If you determine you can treat the wound, you first need to stop the bleeding. You can do this very quickly with a product like Quick Clot or Pet Clot. Clot-producing products work on people as well as pets. These are simple to use. They are packaged as a sponge or gauze pad that you apply to the wound. With a little pressure, the bleeding will stop. Once you have stopped the bleeding and have determined that the wound is one you can treat properly, you can apply medication, such as a triple antibiotic ointment, and bandage the wound if possible. It can be a challenge to keep bandages in place. Animals often remove a bandage faster than you can put it on.

Quick Clot or Pet Clot can be purchased online. Simply type the name in the search line of your preferred Internet search engine, and retailers will pop up. One such website is www.quikclot.com.

PREVENTION

The best prevention, in my opinion, is to keep control of the pet when the pet is outside, such as using a leash when walking the dog or letting the cat out. My experience is that the most severe bleeding is due to the pet being hit by a passing car. Obviously there are other ways that pets can be cut. It is important that sharp objects be put away—and that you are aware of trauma areas within your neighborhood. Pet supervision prevents pet accidents. Take the time—and you will be glad you did.

HAIR STAIN CAUSED BY EYE DISCHARGE

Many dogs have a discolored hair problem from eye discharge at the corner of the eye by the nose. This is seldom seen in cats. The syndrome is frequently seen in Maltese terriers and toy poodles. It tends to be most obvious in small white-haired dogs that have a brown or reddish-brown stain on the hairs along both sides of the nose due to the eye discharge.

The basis of the tearing needs to be investigated since it can be caused by many different syndromes. The lower eyelid could be rolling inward and rubbing on the eyeball, or eyelashes could be poking the eye. Either will cause tearing. Other defects might include nasal folds that interfere with the eye or eyelids, and allergies need to be considered as a culprit. Perhaps the duct that runs from the eye into the nose, which allows excess tears to be discharged into the nose, may be plugged and is not allowing tears to be properly drained into the nose.

This duct is most often called the *nasal lacrimal duct*. In many cases, no specific cause for this problem can be determined. If a condition can be identified, it can be surgically corrected or treated (perhaps as an allergy or obstructed nasal lacrimal duct). Correction of identified defects in or around the eye will normally eliminate tearing, allowing the hairs to be free of staining and tears.

TREATMENT

Affected animals should not be bred. During the past several years, limiting breeding has reduced the incidence of this syndrome. If a defect has been identified and can be corrected, the pet often requires surgery. There is not much that can be done to eliminate the hair staining from tears if the cause of tear production is not identified.

There is a product called Angels' Eyes for dogs and cats that has been used to supposedly remove tear stains. I cannot vouch for the effectiveness of the product since I have not used it. It can be found at online drug sales companies; one company that has the product is 1-800-Pet Meds.

PREVENTION

There is not any known home hair staining prevention currently available. If you have a pet with hair staining syndrome, the basis of the tearing is either treatable or unidentifiable—and most likely not treatable. Both treatable and unidentifiable conditions are normally congenital or developmental.

Due to the way the tearing develops, it unfortunately makes owner prevention unattainable. Eliminating affected dogs from breeding seems to be the best option. Breeding selection has been responsible for greatly reducing the numbers of occurring cases of hair staining due to tears, making this the most effective program for elimination of tear hair stains.

CLEANING EARS

It is easy for you to clean your pet's ears. All you need is a bit of mineral oil and some warm water. Fill the ears with mineral oil and massage vigorously. Let the pet shake its head to get as much of the mineral oil out as possible. Repeat this process three times, being sure to massage the filled ears and letting the pet shake its head.

After you have completed this, fill the ears with warm water and massage the ear. Let the pet shake its head and repeat the water step at least two times. This helps remove the oil from the ears. I have done this on an awful lot of dogs and found that if I use the mineral oil at least three times and the water twice, this procedure will clean ears quite well. This is not 100 percent effective, but at least 80 percent effective. The good news is that the cleaning process can be repeated if necessary.

Due to the head shaking, it is best to do this outdoors or in an area that oil will not get on the new white couch or chair. Just be aware that mineral oil has an oil base and can stain furniture. WaterPiks are great for cleaning ears as well. All that is needed is an old WaterPik and warm water. If this tool is used, try cutting the tip to a straight tip end, which is helpful for cleaning the ears. If you use a WaterPik, remember that you would not want a hard plastic tool jammed into your ear—do not do so to your pet's ear. Be gentle. Sometimes it takes a maximum pressure setting on the WaterPik to clean the ears. Using the lowest pressures will provide the best ear cleaning for your pet. You can adjust the pressures as necessary to complete the ear cleaning.

IS IT ATOPIC SKIN?

Atopy is considered to be an allergen disease that requires treatment by the pet's doctor. This discussion will acquaint you with this complicated, persistent, frustrating skin condition. The condition unfortunately is a skin disease that is not all that uncommon.

An atopic skin condition or so-called atopic dermatitis (AD) is a skin condition that is not caused by skin parasites or fungi; it is an allergy manifested in the skin of dogs and cats. Depending upon the severity of the condition, a pet may scratch and bite at its body. These signs are an indication that the cause of the skin problem needs to be determined. After a visit to the pet's doctor's office—if skin scrapes and other diagnostic tests for skin disease parasites and fungi are not found to be the cause of the skin condition—it becomes a skin allergy issue. When all these normal problems are ruled out, an allergic response needs to be considered.

There are many things that can cause an allergy. Therefore, the diagnosis becomes a challenge to pinpoint the specific dietary or other types of allergens as causative agents for the skin disease. Oh, what the heck, how can it be worse? But it is. The waters become muddier as the skin condition could be atopic-like dermatitis (ALD). You may be asking, "What the heck is this?"

So what is the difference between atopic dermatitis and atopic-like dermatitis? *Canine atopic dermatitis* is used to describe a genetically predisposed itchy inflammatory (pruritic skin) disease that is associated with antibodies (so-called IgE) often due to environmental allergies. It could be seasonal when different allergies are in the air. Canine *atopic-like dermatitis* (ALD) looks and feels like atopic dermatitis, but it has no response to antibodies (IgE) that can be found and documented by environmental allergens. Atopy is thought to be the second most common cause of allergies of cats. Oh boy—what next? You can imagine a cartoon that pictures dollar bills with wings flying away. I realize it is an expense.

Atopy or atopic skin conditions in cats is an exaggerated response to one or more environmental allergens. The allergens are thought to be absorbed into the skin or inhaled. The appearance of this in dogs is red skin on the feet and ears. There may be scratching and biting with this condition. In cats, there may be patchy hair loss over the body associated with scratching and biting at the skin. Skin conditions can be localized or generalized and all over the body.

It is important that fleas be controlled well before jumping off the deep end and looking for other skin conditions. It is very frustrating to spend lots of money trying to get a skin problem diagnosed and solved—and the condition turns out to be fleas. It is always best to get fleas under control, and there are newer and better flea meds on the market than ever before that do a good job eliminating fleas.

Food allergies can be the chief allergy problem, and special diets may be in order to rule out food allergies. Chicken and rice, lamb and rice, and others may be tried. There are many over-the-counter diets at pet stores. An issue with these over-the-counter allergy-preventing diets that produce skin allergies may be a result of the cleaning process of the grinding equipment used to make the food. The manufacturer might mix a regular diet for animals and then clean the equipment and start on an allergy-free diet. The diet can be contaminated due to poor cleaning processes at the manufacturer facility. What you think is an allergen-free diet may not be so, but it is worth a shot. There is no way for you to know that allergy diet feed is contaminated, but you need to be aware of this problem. It has been found to be an issue with pet allergies in over-the-counter foods.

TREATMENT
The condition of atopic skin conditions in dogs and cats is thought to be inherited. Therefore, animals with atopic diseases should not be bred. Treatment of this frustrating and never-ending disease is best left to your pet's doctor since the medications needed to treat the condition are not available over the counter.

PREVENTION
The disease, being an inherited disease, makes preventing it rather unmanageable. If one is lucky, it may just be a seasonal disease and limited to a period of time in the year. The unfortunate will have a year of issues; sometimes a new environment has fewer allergies and may benefit the dog or cat.

MY PET IS LOSING ITS HAIR

Hair loss is common for dogs and cats. This is most often referred to as *alopecia*, which means hair loss. Hair loss always has some issue attached to the reason the hair is disappearing from the skin. The cause can be so-called physiologic hair loss, which can be due to normal hair shedding, or hereditary, as it occurs in some animal breeds. Hair loss can be due to some underlying disease process. Hair loss frequently is not associated with scratching or biting at the skin, which is perhaps most common with dogs and cats that have this problem. Sometimes the pattern of hair loss can be a clue about the cause. Then again, it might not be a clue at all since this is the nature of hair loss in dogs and cats.

Hair loss on the body of animals has four common presentations. One is a generalized hair loss or so-called *diffuse* hair loss. This hair loss is all over the entire body of the pet. Another common finding is a relatively large area of hair loss in a designated area of the body—for example, on a leg, the head, anterior to the tail head (tail head is where the tail attaches to its body), or down the back legs. We refer to this as a *regional* hair loss since it seems to cover a region or area of the body.

On the other hand, the signs present may be patchy, and the patches of hair loss are seen in many spots on the pet's body. They may seem to be everywhere. However, if not generalized, it is in small, multiple patches. We can call this type of hair loss *multifocal*. There is also hair loss where a small patch is only in one spot. This hair loss is referred to as *focal* hair loss. To sum it all up, there are four common patterns of hair loss: *diffuse, regional, multifocal,* and *focal.* Each pattern allows for a clear description of the hair loss, and each can—and most often does—have different causes. Hair loss can also be the result of the same causes and result in different hair patterns. These terms allow a good, simple description of the type of hair loss present on the pet.

Sometimes hair-loss patterns give a clue about the cause of the hair loss. For example, hair loss anterior to the tail head is most often flea allergy dermatitis. This is not to say that this diagnosis is always flea allergy dermatitis. It is most often flea allergy dermatitis, but it could be due to another cause. Hair-loss pattern is not necessarily a diagnostic tool for deciding what disease process is present, but it can be an aid or a suggestion about the underlying cause of the skin disease. For instance, demodex mites can cause focal hair loss or multifocal, diffuse, and regional hair loss. Since demodex mites can be a cause of all hair-loss patterns, they require careful and correct diagnosis so one knows what drug to use to cure the problem.

TREATMENT

There are grocery lists of diseases and metabolic conditions that can cause hair loss with many different hair-loss patterns. These many causes are not a topic of discussion for this issue. However, these hair losses can be broken down into two generalized categorizes— primary and secondary. Due to the complexity of so many skin disease conditions, diagnosis is best left to your pet's favorite doctor.

PREVENTION

With all skin conditions, it is always advisable to make sure you have fleas under control before jumping headlong into other possibilities for hair loss. Fleas can be treated with Advantage II or Advantix II available at pet stores, most Walmart stores, and PX and BX facilities. Normal flea treatment is once every month. The best option for skin issues is to have a preventive medicine program in place for your pet's overall health.

HOT SPOT SKIN INFECTIONS

A hot spot is a terminology used to designate an acute moist skin infection. This condition has also been called *acute moist dermatitis* and *pyotraumatic dermatitis*. Regardless of the name of the condition, it appears quickly. The lesion can be small or very large. Infected areas can be very painful lesions on the skin. This condition is most common in dogs; it is very unusual in cats, but it can occur.

The leading cause of hot spots is not treating for fleas. There are other factors that can be involved, such as associated atopic skin disease of dogs and immune disease conditions. Both origins are rare, however.

One sees more hot spots during the peak flea-production periods when the weather is hot and humid. Hot spots are secondary to self-inflected trauma or so-called iatrogenic trauma. A lesion is created when the dog licks, chews, scratches, or rubs an area on the skin. This is due normally to a sensation to scratch or rub due to an area of skin causing an itching feeling, perhaps due to fleas biting. The lesion seems to occur fast and normally will have fluids (weeping serum) being secreted at the wound site causing matting of the hair on top of the wound and often has infectious fluids associated with the lesion. The hot spot can occur anywhere on the body. My experience is that most hot spots are on the upper part of the back and sides of the body. They can actually be anywhere on the body, including the tail, legs, and other areas.

The painfulness of the infected area makes clipping hair more difficult since the dog may attempt to bite due to the pain of the lesion. It should be assumed that the pet will attempt to bite. Before starting to work on the hot spot, you need to be sure to take the necessary steps to prevent a bite from the dog. Clip the hair and wash the lesion. Washing the lesion seems to almost be as beneficial as medication on the hot spots. Once the hair is clipped and the lesion is cleaned, you are ready to start treatment. The good news is that the skin lesions normally respond quickly to treatment.

TREATMENT

After the hot spot is cleaned, apply triple antibiotics ointments with 1 or 2 percent steroids to the wound. Triple antibiotic ointments are available at grocery stores and pharmacies. This should be done at least two times daily; make sure the wound is cleaned very well before applying any ointments. Continue this treatment two times daily until healed. A word about the incompatibility of furniture and ointments—ointments can stain. Be aware of potential problems if ointments are used indoors.

PREVENTION

Since most hot spots are caused by fleas, a good flea-treatment program keeps the hot spots away.

INJECTION-SITE HAIR LOSS

It is not uncommon for hair loss to occur at a site where a subcutaneous injection has been given. It is normally a focal area of hair loss and may be caused by a rabies immunization, tapeworm medication injection (Praziquantel), steroids, or other compounds. There is no way to know that a pet will have such a reaction. Personally, this issue has been seen more often in a spot where flea meds have been put on the pet rather than from a lack of hair due to injections.

The hair loss seems to develop over time—from two to four months after the injection or the administration of flea medications. The lesions may remain small or enlarge. Rarely, a rabies immunization hair-loss reaction may develop as late as five months after the injection. In cats, the hair loss may come with an itching problem with the cat scratching at the area. In addition to hair loss, cats may ulcerate and develop plaque-like nodular lesions.

It is difficult to tell the difference between a local demodex lesion and an injection or flea medication lesion just by looking at the hair loss area. Therefore, a diagnostic skin scrape is necessary to determine if it is demodex or not. The other issue is knowing the immunization history of the pet to determine postinjection times. In some cats, hair in the injection site area grows back in a different color.

TREATMENT

Topical steroid ointments can be applied to the hair-loss area. These ointments are available at grocery stores and pharmacies as 1 or 2 percent steroid ointments. The pet's doctor may have better or more concentrated medications that might be effective in the treatment of this condition.

PREVENTION

There is no way to predict that a pet will have a hair-loss reaction at the site of an injection of the location were flea medications are applied.

INFECTIONS BETWEEN TOES

The most common interdigital issue is a cyst of a toe that may be due to a foreign body of some type causing an abscess wound. If it is a foreign body, the foreign body must be removed before the wound will heal. The problem with foreign bodies is that they migrate; finding the foreign body becomes a fishing issue. These toe cysts can be very difficult for healing to occur and may become a chronic problem for the foot.

This syndrome is an issue with dogs more than with cats. The cysts will normally affect one toe, but there can be multiple toes involved. Most of the time, there is no known cause of the infection of the toe. The toe can be swollen, and it may be draining infectious materials from the toe. The infected toe or toes often cause lameness.

Causes of interdigital cysts can be food allergies, atopy, infected hairs, or hair bristles. Grass awns (sharp, pointed grass seeds) can cause severe problems for dog's toes due to grass awn skin's penetrating and migration abilities. Other common instigators of infected toes include tumors, metabolic causes like hypothyroidism, and a grocery list of others.

If the pet is chewing at the foot, a method of stopping the chewing will need to be found. The best one can do is to use an Elizabethan collar, which is available at pet stores such as Petco and PetSmart. Some cases are so bad that they require surgery for treatment.

The first issue is to determine, if possible, what the cause of the infection is. That can be a real challenge. It may take the expertise of your pet's doctor to determine the best treatment for the digital cyst.

TREATMENT

Most often, the treatment will require systemic antibiotics or other medications and keeping the foot bandaged until the toe heals. Remember that these cysts are a hard wound to heal, and it may take both you and your veterinarian working together to resolve any toe issues your pet may have.

PREVENTION

Often the origin of the toe cyst is unknown. If one is in an area where grass awns or thorns are present, a quick look at the feet for potential foreign bodies is advisable. There is little more that can be done to prevent this syndrome from occurring.

TOENAIL ISSUES

On occasion, there is inflammation of the toenails and other issues with the toenails or the surrounding tissues. One of the more common is a fungal infection of the toes and toenails. Fungal infections may cause the toenails to be brittle—causing them to break easily—or the toenails to be sloughed off and creating a deformity of the toenails. The kinds of fungus infections may vary between dogs and cats, but the treatment of either kind of fungus can be treated with the same medication.

Toenails may be traumatized in one way or another, causing the toenails to break or even be torn away, resulting in bleeding from the toenail. The bleeding can be stopped by putting cornstarch on the bleeding toenail.

There are many other causes of toenail issues, but most are not common. Some examples of other toenail issues are cancer of the foot or toes, immune mediated diseases, bacterial infections, yeast infections, autoimmune diseases, and fungal infections. Parasites, such as demodex, are perhaps the top toenail-causing issues that might be seen in the toes of dogs and cats. Rest assured that there can be other causes not mentioned here.

TREATMENT

Bleeding toenails due to trauma or toenail trimming can be stopped with cornstarch. If one is about to trim toenails, it is a good idea to get the cornstarch out before starting the nail trim. As for fungal infections of the toes, there is a need to have a proper diagnosis so an appropriate treatment can be initiated.

What might look like a fungal infection may be bacterial. It is better that your pet's doctor diagnoses the toenail problem and gives you the cause of the toenail problem. The pet's doctor may also dispense oral antifungal drugs that will help the toes heal much faster. If it is a fungus in the tissues around the toenail, it is possible that it can be treated with Tinactin or other over-the-counter topical fungal medications. If the fungal infection is within the toenail, no topical treatment will be effective. This type of toenail infection requires oral medicating before it will be effective. You will need medications or a prescription from your pet's doctor to obtain the proper systemic medication treatment.

PREVENTION
Keeping your pet clean and frequently checking the animal—and having your pet's doctor check via the wellness program—is perhaps the best one can do to aid in the health of the pet's feet. Catching issues early is a method for successful treatment and the prevention of advanced disease conditions. This attention to detail keeps veterinary costs low when compared to treatments of disease conditions.

SKIN YEAST INFECTION (MALASSEZIA)

The bad news is that skin yeast infections are rather common in dogs and cats. The disease is difficult to treat in order to get a good healing of the infected skin. The yeast can be on the bottom of the chest and belly, on and in the ears, or on the lips. The lip infections are caused from licking at the infected skin. The reasons that the skin condition occurs are not completely understood. It may be related to allergies, skin oil secretions, poor skin development, congenital skin development, or hormones. The condition in cats is rare, but it does occur and can be as bad as skin yeast infections in dogs.

Often there is a rather intense itching sensation resulting in lots of biting, licking, and scratching at the infected area. Not all pets seem to have the same intensity of the itching sensation. The skin may be wrinkled, look like elephant skin, or have a dark (almost black) appearance. Other times, it is gray and looks like scaling skin.

In addition to the yeast presence, there is normally a secondary invasion of bacteria. The skin is made of cells—each cell has a membrane or wall around the cell. Within each cell there are intracellular organelles and materials present. If the pet has a skin-yeast infection (malassezia), the cells of the skin will appear as if the cell walls are missing, which will allow the intracellular materials of the cells to bunch together. The condition is often helped with the treatment of omega-3 fatty acids and is often suggested as an adjunct to the yeast infection.

There is an odor that is associated with the condition; once it is identified, you will recognize it if the opportunity happens to arise. Unfortunately, if treatment is successful, the condition often comes roaring right back.

TREATMENT

The medications necessary for the treatment of these conditions are not available over the counter. To add to the frustration, treatment of this normally chronic and seemingly never-healing condition is best handled by the pet's doctor. You perhaps can aid the skin condition by administering omega-3 fatty acids. Treatment will usually require antifungal medication and antibiotics among other drugs necessary to control the skin yeast infection.

PREVENTION

There are a lot of unknowns with this skin disease, and it may be an inherited condition. The pet should not be bred. Certainly if it can be identified early, it may be prevented or stopped from becoming much worse when it will be very difficult to treat. This is another great reason to consider establishing a wellness program with your favorite veterinarian.

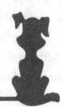

CHAPTER 2

MY PET IS SICK (DISEASES)

If you find yourself in a hole, stop digging.
—Will Rogers

A medical definition of disease is "an interruption, cessation, or disorder of body functions, systems, or organs." Volumes have been written on diseases. In the early days, there were four components of disease: phlegm, black bile, yellow bile, and blood; if these elements fell out of balance, the patient became sick. We have come a long way, baby. Thank goodness.

Disease can mean a lot of different issues for pets. Diseases could be from bacteria, viruses, rickets, nutrition, or tumors. The goal is to prevent any disease from occurring; in this millennium, we recognize that prevention is the best method of defense. The bad news is that diseases occur, and they need to be treated. The body will not always be able to defeat the bad guys, which are the germs, etc.

In this chapter, many diseases are presented that pets can get. You may be able to treat them at home, but some will require the aid of the pet's doctor. This chapter also contains methods to stop the disease from occurring in the first place; prevention is the goal. Most often prevention is very simple. We as people tend to ignore simple pet health preventive measures (steps, or programs), but in health it means money out of pocket and in some cases death.

SHOULD I TREAT MY PET OR PUT IT DOWN?

Unfortunately, there is no simple answer for this common question. Many pets have become so attached to us that it becomes a very emotional problem for owners to decide. Should I go for broke or let go?

The first determinant should be whether the pet has a chance of being well. Will the pet have a palatable quality of life without being healed? Second is the financial concern. How much can you afford? It is not a lack of love for the pet—but what can the pocketbook afford. As an example, our cat had a small thyroid tumor. The choice was several thousand dollars for radiation therapy or surgery. The doctor was not comfortable doing the surgery, but we opted for surgery since the cost was $300 for surgery instead of $4,000 for radiation. This is a common everyday experience and concern in the real world. The cat with surgery lived about four more years.

The next issue is the excruciating process of making a medical decision one knows that he or she needs to make involving the life of the pet. The decision is so emotional that most often the wrong decision is made. I have friends who call to get a second opinion for their pet. I do not give a direct answer, but I explain several cases that are similar. I have no pixie dust to tell people a magic answer. I relate similar cases. I have had cases in which the people spent money they really could not afford and later had to put the pet down.

As an example of wrong decisions due to emotion, a friend with an ill pet asked for my advice. I recommended putting the pet down. He opted to treat; after thousands of dollars, he put the pet down. Later he said, "I should have listened to you." This illustrates the difficulty in the decision-making process that one has to go through.

TREATMENT

The bottom line is that each pet owner has to be the one to make the final decision. No one can make up your mind or make the decision for you. You have to make the decision. Others can suggest things, but they are only suggestions. A problem a pet owner can have is getting the heart and brain on the same page. When one arrives at this point, it allows one to start thinking of the pet's quality of life instead of your own deep, loving feelings. It is hard to think about quality instead of quantity in these very stressful situations.

PREVENTION

There, of course, is no prevention. There is no way to tell what health experiences any living organism will experience.

ELEVATED TEMPERATURES IN CATS AND DOGS

On occasion, you may believe that your pet is not doing well. One of the first things you can do is take the temperature of your pet. This is a rather simple process, and any thermometer can be used to obtain the temperature. An old glass thermometer or a digital thermometer will do; the brand or type makes no difference as long as it will record the temperature.

The best way to obtain the temperature of your pet is to lubricate the end of the thermometer with an ointment. Make sure the ointment does not cause a burning sensation, such as Vicks. You can use products such as K-Y jelly, Vaseline, or similar products. The lubricant will make it easier to place the thermometer into the anus.

With the old type of thermometers, it will take about one to two minutes to obtain an accurate temperature. Modern digital thermometers will record the temperature in a few seconds, but they cost considerably more. Normal temperatures for a dog range from 100.5 to 102.5 degrees Fahrenheit. If the dog is outside on a hot day, a normal temperature can be as high as 103.5 degrees Fahrenheit. Any higher is considered an elevated temperature in a dog.

A cat's normal temperature ranges from 100.4 to 102.5 degrees Fahrenheit. Sometimes a pet will allow one person to take a temperature. However, most often you will need another person to help you take the temperature of your pet—one to hold the pet and one to take the temperature. Remember when using an older thermometer, you need to shake it until the thermometer reads a low number, such as below 90 degrees.

To get the temperature of your pet, raise the tail and insert the lubricated thermometer slowly into the rectum [anus], which is located just below the tail. Insert the thermometer about an inch or so and hold in place about two minutes for the old-style mercury thermometer or until you hear a beep for the more-modern digital thermometer. Remove the thermometer and read the temperature. Remember a temperature below normal can be just as serious as an elevated temperature.

Be assured that you cannot determine the temperature of a pet by feeling the skin of an animal or the ears, nose, or head. The skin and other parts of the body can feel warm to your touch and may have a normal temperature—or your pet could have an elevated temperature. The only way to know if a pet's temperature is elevated is to use a thermometer.

Some common signs that *might* accompany an elevated temperature in a pet are lethargy, weakness, unwillingness to move, lack of appetite, and dehydration. You will note that these signs are similar to a lot of other health conditions, and the signs will not give you any clue about the cause of an elevated temperature. Many elevated temperatures are not correlated to any known risk factors.

Causes of elevated temperatures range from simple to complex—excitement, small skin wounds, abscesses, injury from trauma (such as smashed muscles or broken bones, kidney infections, immune-mediated diseases, tumors, viral or fungal infections, and even some medications).

Many pets may have what is called fever of unknown origin (FUO). Please note that none are treatable by you, and many will require a complete blood count, blood chemistry, or other tests for pancreatitis, lupus, and immune-mediated arthritis. However, you will know that your pet has an issue and needs to see the pet's doctor.

I encourage you to examine your pet frequently. If you are interested in doing so, there are useful guidelines on how to examine your pet in *How to Treat Your Dogs and Cats with Over-the-Counter Drugs Companion Edition.* There are several pages at the back of this book to record your pet's temperatures and other data every time you examine your pet.

TREATMENT

There are so many different causes of elevated temperature; it is difficult to know if an antibiotic or painkiller would be best for the pet. I believe strongly that elevated temperatures need the diagnostic capability and medical assistance of the pet's doctor.

I know that many folks will give some type of medication to their pet regardless of what I think or say. Realizing this, the following aspirin charts (Table 2.1) are provided for both cats and dogs. I am reluctant to provide this information since many folks have used excessive amounts of aspirin and compounded or caused death or illness. Table 2.1 provides aspirin dosage according to your pet's weight. Find your pet's weight in the chart to obtain the correct amount for your pet. *Do not overdose.* Aspirin can be purchased at grocery stores, pharmacies, Walmart, and pet stores.

PREVENTION

The best thing you can do is consider a wellness program with your pet's doctor and plan on a least two pet visits with the doctor each year. You can practice giving your pet physical exams (see *How to Treat Your Dogs and Cats with Over-the-Counter Drugs Companion Edition,* p. 31–38) so you will have recorded data when the pet is healthy. This data will help you know when there is a deviation from normal. If you do not know your pet's normal values, you will not know when there is a disease deviation.

Table 2.1 Dog Aspirin Dosage

Aspirin is not recommended for cats.
Use enteric-coated aspirin.

Caution Special Notice: Due to the availability of aspirin in only 81 and 325 mg tablets, it is impossible to be accurate with dosage. Dosing is ballpark dose because you have to cut the tablets into quarters or halves. For safety, any pet less than five pounds should have a prescription. For pain meds from the pet's doctor, give every twelve hours.

Weight Pounds	Low Dose 4.5 mg /lb. 81 mg Tablet	High Dose 11 mg / lb. 325 mg Tablet	Weight Pounds	Low Dose 4.5 mg /lb. 325 mg Tablet	High Dose 11 mg / lb. 325 mg Tablet	Weight Pounds	Low Dose 4.5 mg /lb. 325 mg Tablet	High Dose 11 mg / lb. 325 mg Tablet
5	.25	.25	26	.25	1	46	.75	1+.5
6	.25	.25	27	.25	1	47	.75	1+.5
7	.25	,25	28	.25	1	48	.75	1+.5
8	.5	.25	29	.25	1	49	.75	1+.5
9	.5	.25	30	.5	1	50	.75	1+.75
10	.5	.25	31	.5	1	51	.75	1+.75
11	.5	.5	31	.5	1	52	.75	1+.75
12	.5	.5	33	.5	1+.25	53	.75	1+.75
13	.75	.5	34	.5	1+.25	54	.75	2
14	.75	.5	35	.5	1+.25	55	.75	2
15	.75	.5	36	.5	1+.25	56	.75	2
16	.75	.5	37	.5	1+.25	57	.75	2
17	1	.5	38	.5	1+.25	58	.75	2
18	1	.5	39	.5	1+.25	59	.75	2
19	1	.75	40	.5	1+.5	60	.75	2
20	1	.75	41	.5	1+.5	61	.75	2
	Low Dose 4.5 mg/ lb. 325 mg Tablet							
21	.25	.75	42	.5	1+.5	62	.75	2
22	.25	.75	43	.5	1+.5	63	1	2
23	.25	.75	44	.5	1+.5	64	1	2
24	.25	.75	45	.5	1+.5	65	1	2

Weight Pounds	Low Dose 4.5 mg /lb. 325 mg Tablet	High Dose 11 mg / lb. 325 mg Tablet	Weight Pounds	Low Dose 4.5 mg /lb. 325 mg Tablet	High Dose 11 mg / lb. 325 mg Tablet	Weight Pounds	Low Dose 4.5 mg /lb. 325 mg Tablet	High Dose 11 mg / lb. 325 mg Tablet
66	1	2+.25	78	1	2+.75	90	1+.25	3
67	1	2+.25	79	1	2+.75	91	1+.25	3+.25
68	1	2+.25	80	1+.25	2+.75	92	1+.25	3+.25
69	1	2+.25	81	1+.25	2+.75	93	1+.25	3+.25
70	1	2+.5	82	1+.25	2+.75	94	1+.25	3+.25
71	1	2+.5	83	1+.25	2+.75	95	1+.25	3+.25
72	1	2+.5	84	1+.25	3	96	1+.25	3+.25
73	1	2+.5	85	1+.25	3	97	1+.25	3+.25
74	1	2+.5	86	1+.25	3	98	1+.5	3+.25
75	1	2+.5	87	1+.25	3	99	1+.5	3+.25
76	1	2+.5	88	1+.25	3	100	1+.5	3+.5
77	1	2+.5	89	1+.25	3			

Table 2.2 *Cat Aspirin Dosage*

Aspirin 81 mg Tablet

Low dose give 4.5 mg/ pound every seventy-two hours.
High dose give 4.5 mg / pound every forty-eight hours.

Special Note: Dosage is approximate due to the need to cut tablets.

Weight Pounds	Low Dose Tablet or Parts of Tablet to Be Given Every 72 Hours	High Dose Tablet or Parts of Tablet to Be Given Every 48 Hours	Weight Pounds	Low Dose Tablet or Parts of Tablet to Be Given Every 72 Hours	High Dose Tablet or Parts of Tablet to Be Given Every 48 Hours
1	Too small	Too small	11	.5 + .12 Or ½ + 1/8	.5 + .12 Or ½ + 1/8
2	Too small	Too small	12	.5 + .12 or ½ + 1/8	.5 + .12 or ½ + 1/8
3	Too small	Too small	13	¾ or .75	½+1/4 or .75
4	¼ or .25	¼ or .25	14	¾ or .75	½+1/4 or .75
5	¼ or .25	¼ or .25	15	¾ + 1/8 Or .75 .12	½+1/4 + 1/8 or .75 .12
6	¼ + 1/8 or .25 +.12	¼ + 1/8 or .25 +.12	16	¾ + 1/8 Or .75 + .12	¾ + 1/8 or .75 +.12
7	.25 + .12 or ¼ + 1/8	.25 + .12 or ¼ + 1/8	17	1	1
8	½ or .5	½ or .5	18	1	1
9	½ or .5	½ or .5	19	1	1
10	½ or .5	½ or .5	20	1 = 1/8 or 1 + .12	1 = 1/8 or 1 + .12

Parts of the aspirin 1/8 = .12, ¼ = .25, ½ = .5, ½ + ¼ = ¾ or .75, lbs. = pounds

- mg per 1/8 or .12 of a tablet = 10 mg
- mg per ¼ or .25 of a tablet = 20 mg
- mg per ½ or .5 of tablet of a tablet = 40 mg
- mg per ½ + ¼ = ¾ or .75 of a tablet = 60 mg
- mg per 1 tablet = 81 mg

FELINE LEUKEMIA VIRUS INFECTION (FELV)

Feline Leukemia Virus, more commonly noted by the acronym of FeLV, is a cat disease that is more common in cats in the outside and young cats less than a year old. Interestingly, it is found most often in domestic feral cats, which may be due to the social living of cats as they do not share with other wild animals.

Feral cats often stay within a colony of other cats in the wild. It is the free-roaming cats that are most likely to be infected; a housecat that is never let out is very unlikely to become infected. However, if the cat is allowed to go outside or gets out of the house accidentally, the cat can become infected due to association with other cats in the outside environments. For example, if you or a neighbor feeds or waters feral cats, which is very common, and your cat happens to eat or drink from those containers, your indoor-outdoor cat can become infected with FeLV.

Catfights are a common way of spreading the disease since bites transmit saliva along with the gift of an FeLV infection—in addition to the added benefits of abscess-causing bacterial infections.

FeLV is spread through saliva—not the respiratory system. It is spread by sharing food and water bowls, grooming, blood transfusions, or transplacentally. In fact, it has been demonstrated that sharing litter with an infected cat can spread the disease in the feces. It is not a contagious disease or spread by contact—and it is *not* zoonotic or spread to people.

Environmental contamination is of a lesser concern due to the fact that the virus is highly sensitive and is very rapidly destroyed or killed due to desiccation, disinfectants, and heat. FeLV is found worldwide, but there seems to be a worldwide decrease in the prevalence of the disease (possibly due to the results of test and removal and vaccination programs).

PREVENTION

The best prevention is to keep the cat or cats in the house and not let them out. This approach is often referred to as isolation. The next best thing to do is to test for FeLV, followed by immunizing the pet. A pound of prevention is worth a ton of treatment, and it saves big dollars for you.

This brings up a thought about immunizations. If you are concerned about adjuvant vaccines, you need to know that some FeLV vaccines can be adjuvanted. Nonadjuvanted recombinant FeLV vaccines are also available. Vaccinating against FeLV is not considered a core vaccine, but it is recommended for cats at risk of exposure, indoor-outdoor cats, or cats living with known infected cats. The concern about adjuvanted vaccines is the formation of tumors with any adjuvanted vaccines. The tumor-formation reaction seems to be linked genetically for some cats.

CAT AIDS OR FELINE IMMUNODEFICIENCY DISEASE

Cat AIDS is called FIV or Feline Immunodeficiency Virus. FIV has a prevalence of less than 5 percent in the North American cat population (owned and feral). Feline immunodeficiency is often confused with FeLV. FeLV has declined over the past few years, mostly due to removing infected cats. However, the infection rate of FIV has remained at a rather constant infectious rate within the North American cat population.

FIV is a species- or cat-specific disease and poses no apparent risk to human populations. The cause of the disease was discovered in 1986 by Dr. Neals Pederson of the College of Veterinary Medicine at the University of California–Davis. It was isolated from a cattery at that time. It has remained a research interest ever since it was discovered and continues to this day.

Bite wounds are the major source of infection of FIV among cats. There is evidence that cats that live in close proximity to each other over a period of time may become infected. It has been surmised that saliva from sharing food and water dishes may be a source of this type of infection. There are those who suggest that using the same litter box may be a source of infection for cats living in close proximity.

Female cats that become infected during pregnancy will transmit the disease in utero and in the first milk (colostrum). Though not common, it will cause newborn kittens to be infected at birth. Male cats that are allowed to roam free commonly become infected due to their fighting instincts or behavior. Kittens not born with FIV are not any more susceptible to FIV than adult cats are. However, kittens are not normally infected with FIV.

TREATMENT

Treatments for FIV are normally beyond the capability of doing it yourself since most are system types of treatments for which you lack the diagnostic capability and treatment capability. This is best left to the judgment of your pet's doctor; treatment plans and recommendations may include euthanasia.

PREVENTION

Vaccinations are available for FIV disease, and are the best and easiest prevention you can provide for your cat or cats. The vaccine is for cats eight weeks of age or older, and it is recommended that the cat receive a series of three immunizations given at two- or three-week intervals and annually after the initial three immunizations. Prevention is by far the cheapest and best solution for any disease—and especially for diseases such as FIV for which we currently have no treatment.

FREQUENT SQUATTING AND NOTHING HAPPENS

This seems to be a common observation of pets by owners. Frequent squatting most commonly is due to a urinary tract infection. Many folks seem to think this is a sign of constipation—and it could be. However, the most common cause of this activity in pets is a urinary tract infection.

This condition is not normally treatable by owners of pets due to the need to obtain an accurate diagnosis and medication that will treat the infection in the urinary tract. This information is provided because this is a frequent observation of pet owners. Urinary tract infections can become very serious in a short period of time if not properly cared for.

TREATMENT

The good news is that most urinary tract infections can normally be treated very effectively if the pet is started on antibiotics. It is best when an infection is caught early. When the first signs are noticed, it is prudent to take your pet to the pet's favorite doctor—and the sooner, the better. Delay most often allows more stubborn infections to become established.

PREVENTION

Perhaps the best program of prevention is a good, well-established preventive medicine program that you can set up with the pet's doctor for a semiannual checkup with blood and urinary systems tests. These tests will ensure that your pet's health is stable and will pick up bad health conditions early if they happen to be noted at a routine checkup.

I have been asked if it is necessary to go to the veterinarian when the pet seems to be doing okay. My answer is that my physician sees me routinely every six months; there have been times when he picked up issues early, which prevented further development of the noted findings. A wellness program is much better than doing nothing—and a heck of a lot cheaper than treating any medical issues. My answer to the question is absolutely yes—having a wellness program is the best you can do for your pet buddy.

DRINKING EXCESSIVE WATER AND FREQUENT URINATION

There are many things that can cause a pet to drink lots of water, and most are due to a systemic disease that takes testing to determine the cause. One of the common causes is due to a urinary tract infection. When excessive amounts of liquids are consumed, it will normally cause excessive urination. If a pet is squatting a lot—and there seems to be no discharge—it is often due to an infection of the bladder or the urinary tract.

The bad news is that excessive drinking and urination are not normal. In most cases, this will require the pet's doctor to run tests to determine the origins of this syndrome. Some other disease conditions that might bring on excessive water consumption and urination are renal failure, overproduction of steroids by the adrenal glands (hyperadrenocorticism), urinary tract infections, and diabetes mellitus in dogs. In cats, the origin might be hyperthyroidism, renal failure, urinary tract infections, or diabetes mellitus. All require tests that the pet's doctor can run.

TREATMENT

Unfortunately, the condition of excessive water consumption and frequent urination (more commonly called *polydipsia* and *polyuria*) are a job for your pet's veterinarian. The testing equipment availability at home is nonexistent, and the machines are extremely expensive. Also, the technology is way beyond the instrumentation and capability of home treatments.

PREVENTION

The problem with these two issues is that they might be in the process of starting when the pet seems normal, but the signs appear gradually. After it starts, the increases are not noticeable until it becomes advanced. When you put more water in the bowl, it becomes apparent that something is wrong. These conditions alone justify the need for a wellness program with your favorite veterinary practice. These are some conditions that will be caught early with such a program.

LICK DERMATITIS OF DOGS

This is a tough nut to crack, and it is a frequent problem in dogs. Dogs will lick and chew and lick and lick at one particular spot on the body. It seems to be more on the front legs, but the rear legs are not exempt by any means. In the area where they lick, lesions develop. These lick granulomas probably should be called *frustrating granulomas.* The name granuloma is due to the type of tissues that develop due to traumatized skin caused by licking at a particular spot all the time.

Too bad there is not some pixie dust to sprinkle on this, but there is frustration after frustration trying to resolve this type of issue for your pet. This one is definitely a frustration you can push onto your pet's doctor so he or she can be frustrated too. Many of these lick dermatitis problems are chronic and reoccurring. Many things have been tried. All of the trying has caused learning in the same tradition as Thomas Edison. Thomas Edison found a thousand things that would not work during his frustrating trials to invent the light bulb. Alas, the famous lick dermatitis of dogs is in the same ballpark.

There are supposed to be a lot of things that cause this syndrome, such as demodex skin mites. At our facility, we get demodex dogs coming out of our ears—and not a single dog has lick dermatitis. They might have demodex, but it sure as heck is a very rare cause of granuloma.

Other doctors suspect the following to be causes of lick granuloma: fungal infections, foreign bodies, degenerative joint disease, pressure point granuloma, and calcium deposits in the skin. In my forty years as a practicing veterinarian I have never seen any correlation among the preceding conditions and lick granuloma. This is not to say there is no correlation, only that it is rare. Boredom is the number-one cause of lick granuloma—a bored dog licks and licks. It is better to be proactive rather than reactive. The best preventive measure for lick granuloma is exercising the dog and avoiding long periods of confinement. Pet isolation seems to create the perfect-storm setting for lick granuloma.

TREATMENT

This frustration rightly belongs to the dog's doctors; they might have an answer and solve the problem of the lick granuloma. If they do, take them a bag of M&M's for solving your dog's granuloma and say, "Thank God you did it."

PREVENTION

This one is endemic, and it happens when it happens, but if a dog is bored, you probably have the stage set for a lick dermatitis or granuloma. Get the dog out and let it run. Tire it out so it sleeps and then run the dog some more to keep it active. Do not give it a chance to be bored. I believe a farm is the place for a lick dermatitis dog so it has space to run.

CATS AND PLASTIC FEEDING DISHES

I hesitate to discuss this topic because I have no proof or scientific studies to prove what I am about to write. However, many cat owners and cat rescue people have told me that they have observed the comments that follow. I know that using plastic bowls for feeding and watering dogs can cause an allergic reaction to the lips that can be so bad that the lips are bright red and ooze serum due to the reaction to the plastic dishes. I have seen this in dogs and treated the condition with great success by switching the dishes to ceramic, glass, or metal (prescription steroids helped speed recovery).

The syndrome did not reoccur if plastic feeding dishes were not used for feeding or watering. The signs in dogs are not an all-or-nothing condition, but they seem to affect a certain number of dogs. Perhaps due to genetic makeup of the dog, the allergic response might be compared to a dog's response to an allergy stimulated by pollens. With the dog issue in mind and the comments received from so many cat owners and cat rescue people, I sort of have a basis to believe what I am about to write. Your actions on this issue are your choice since I cannot prove the following. You can try it—you have nothing to lose and perhaps a lot to gain—for your cat problems.

I have been told that using plastic dishes for feeding and watering of cats can cause chin issues, such as blackheads, hair loss, and some other chin issues. I have noted several cats with chin issues—some severe, and others not so bad. At our facility, we have no history of any animal that arrives, and no previous knowledge of the cats observed is known. As with the dog, if this cat allergy to plastic is a true syndrome, then only certain cats would be affected and not 100 percent of the cat population.

Assuming the above is true, the following suggested treatment prevention is provided for your consideration.

TREATMENT

If your cat has chin issues, give this a try. Just stop using plastic dishes to feed and water your cat. Try a glass, ceramic, or metal bowl—and you are the judge of the final results. If your cat has chin sores or hair loss, remember that no medical issue is an overnight cure. I do know if it works for your cat, the cost of the bowls is a lot cheaper than a trip to the veterinary hospital for cat chin problems. It worked when our cat had a small area of hair loss on the chin.

PREVENTION

If the food and water dishes are the problem, switch to ceramic or metal feeding or watering dishes. Cats like to drink out of cups, and any that are not plastic would be fine.

BUBONIC PLAGUE

Yes, this is the same disease that wiped out hundreds of communities and killed millions of people years ago in Europe. The bad news is that this disease is still found in the United States, most often in summer in New Mexico, Arizona, California, Colorado, Idaho, Nevada, Oregon, Texas, Utah, Washington, Wyoming, and Hawaii. However, with the quick traveling population, this disease can easily be transported anywhere in the world. Years ago, heartworm was thought to be limited to certain areas of the country, and today heartworm is everywhere. Do not hang your hat on the idea that this is only a Western issue.

Cats are more frequently infected with this disease than dogs— probably because cats are explorers and need to poke their noses into everything, and they hunt and eat rodents. Some references consider eating plague-diseased rodents as the primary way cats become infected with plague bacteria (*Yersinia pestis*). The other mode of transmitting the disease is by biting fleas.

Dogs are not immune to this disease, but they do not have anywhere near the number of cases as cats. To make it worse for cats, they are very susceptible to infection and catch fatal diseases quickly and exhibit lung or pulmonary and blood infections with the organisms in the bloodstream. The incubation period of the disease is two to seven days after a flea bite or eating an infected rodent.

Cats develop buboes (open, draining sores) on the head and neck; this might be a first sign that the cat has bubonic plague. Under the skin (subcutaneous areas), there can be lumps or enlargements due to infection of the most superficial lymph nodes. Deeper lymph nodes are also infected, but they may not be able to be seen until they burst open and drain thick white pus.

The lymph nodes will develop rapidly and fill with thick white pus (exudates) and burst and expel infected materials. When infected nodes start bursting in the lung tissue, the cat will expel the plague disease in its breath.

The lung form of the disease in cats is very deadly and is not as common as other forms of the disease. A cat may be dead before the lymph nodes have a chance to enlarge and expel the thick white exudates. An infected cat's temperature is often 103–105° F (39.5–40.5° Celsius). There may be vomiting, diarrhea, dehydration, enlarged tonsils, anorexia, eye discharge, weight loss, walking incoordination, coma, and oral ulcers. Some cats may develop the disease without abscess formation but still have the other signs of bubonic plague.

Plague in dogs depends upon how long the dog has had the disease. The dog may be feverish and depressed; as the disease progresses, it becomes worse and may start to show some of the same signs noted in cats. The unfortunate problem is that early signs may be interpreted as bite wounds in dogs and cats.

TREATMENT
This is a reportable disease and should be handled by your pet's doctor. This disease is often transmitted to people. We have antibiotics for

treatment, but this is such a nasty disease that without professional help, it is a disaster. Do not hesitate to seek help. It is most often recommend that the pet be euthanized due to threats to humans.

PREVENTION

The best you can do is to be sure to treat for fleas since a flea bite by an infected flea is as bad as eating an infected rodent. If you have outside cats that come into the house, you may be aware that your cat may bring some of the rodents into the house. The rodent may be infested with fleas, which will contaminate your home. This is not a condition to mess with; it is very deadly. A hair raising fact is that allowing pets to sleep in bed with people has been shown to increase the risk of people getting plague (CDC).

If the rodent brings fleas in the house, your family might become infected with plague. You can take the rodent to your veterinarian and have it checked out, but if you handle such things, you need to be wearing rubber gloves that are disposed of immediately. Remember that any leaking infections are expelling bacteria of *Yersinia pestis* into your environment and will be a threat to your family.

CDC recommends 1. Treat dogs and cats for fleas. 2. Keep pet food in rodent-proof containers 3. Take sick pets to the Pets Doctor 4. Do not allow pet's access to rodent habitats such as prairie dog colonies.

OH NO! MY PET HAS HEARTWORMS

The good news is that you could have prevented heartworms had you put your pet on a heartworm preventive. There are several options that are discussed below under prevention. If your pet has a positive heartworm test, it does not mean that the pet has heartworm disease. Many animals can have a positive heartworm test without the disease effects as a result of the heartworm infection.

If you have a preventive medicine program with your pet's doctor, this condition most likely would have been avoided or at least diagnosed early so there would be no disease development. There is more bad news. Treatment of heartworm disease is very expensive, and prices can range widely. If you are going to have your pet treated, you might want to shop around since treatment prices can vary quite a lot. You might be able to locate a facility that will meet your budgetary needs.

Heartworms are manifested differently in cats than in the dogs. The disease in cats is frequently more prevalent in lung tissues. The juvenile worms tend to die in the bloodstream. These dead worms and/or pieces of dead worms are then distributed into lung blood vessels, causing severe inflammation in the cat's lung tissues. Signs in cats might include coughing, rapid and difficult breathing, and vomiting.

Unfortunately, these signs do not come with a sign that says the cat has heartworms. Therefore, tests are necessary for diagnosing the disease. Seldom do the heartworms live to be adults in cats, but it has happened. Due to the adult heartworms not maturing in cats, they do not normally have the heart conditions that develop in dogs. The heartworm respiratory problems of cats have been identified as heartworm-associated respiratory disease (HARD).

Active dogs develop more severe lesions from heartworm infections then inactive dogs do. Heartworms mature in the bloodstream and in the right side of the heart. The worms in the heart cause the right atrium to enlarge and damage the right heart valve. This creates right heart valve leakage and damage and abnormal right heart sounds.

Heartworms, like all living things, die—and the parts of the dead worms then flow through the blood vessels into the lungs. Over a period of time, this causes considerable blood vessel blockage and infections in the lungs. Signs might include coughing, fatigue, limited activity tolerance, difficulty breathing, coughing up blood, bleeding from the nose, and loss of consciousness. The signs are not specific to heartworm disease, and the diagnosis will require special tests.

When a dog is treated for heartworms, the worms tend to die at about the same time, causing a large amount of worm parts to flow to the lungs and block blood vessels and cause infections. This is partly why treatment is so severe. A pet undergoing treatment should be kept relatively quiet and have limited activity and exercise as directed by the pet's doctor. Lots of activity could kill the pet if the doctor's directions are not followed.

Mosquitoes carry the disease. Mosquitoes can have three and some say 10 heartworm larvae in one mosquito; when they draw blood from a dog or cat, the larvae are injected into the body of the animal. The mosquito picks up the larvae by biting an infected animal, which becomes the host for the parasite.

Meanwhile, the larvae develop through three stages before they can infect other animals. The development in the mosquito depends on the ambient temperature and humidity. The shortest time for development in the mosquito is ten days.

If you are interested, you can go online. In the search option of your search engine, type in American Heartworm Society, and you will be taken to the heartworm website or you can go to http://www. heartwormsociety.org.

TREATMENT

The treatment is best left to your veterinarian. There are different protocols for treatment of heartworms. Therefore, we will not discuss treatment procedures. The protocol used will be explained by your pet's doctor.

PREVENTION

You can easily prevent this disease from occurring in your pet by using the dosage chart below (Table 2.3). The dose of 1 percent Ivermectin is determined by weight of your pet. Look for your pet's weight to obtain the dose to give. Giving the designated dose according to your pet's weight once per month will prevent heartworms—and will treat roundworms, hookworms, and ear mites. It is very important not to overdose your pet. Give only the dose found within the chart according to your pet's weight.

Table 2.3 1 Percent Ivermectin Dose-by-Weight Chart

(weight divided by 80 = dose in cc)
Use for heartworm prevention, nondemodex skin mites,
roundworms, hookworms, whipworms, and Strongyloides.
Do not overdose!

Weight Pounds	Dose cc	Weight Pounds	Dose cc	Weight Pounds	Dose cc	Weight Pounds	Dose cc	Weight Pounds	Dose cc
1	0.01	21	0.26	41	0.51	61	0.76	81	1.01
2	0.02	22	0.27	42	0.52	62	0.77	82	1.02
3	0.03	23	0.28	43	0.53	63	0.78	83	1.03
4	0.05	24	0.30	44	0.55	64	0.80	84	1.05
5	0.06	25	0.31	45	0.56	65	0.81	85	1.06
6	0.07	26	0.32	46	0.57	66	0.82	86	1.07
7	0.08	27	0.33	47	0.58	67	0.83	87	1.08
8	0.10	28	0.35	48	0.60	68	0.85	88	1.10
9	0.11	29	0.36	49	0.61	69	0.86	89	1.11
10	0.12	30	0.37	50	0.62	70	0.87	90	1.12
11	0.13	31	0.38	51	0.63	71	0.88	91	1.13
12	0.15	32	0.40	52	0.65	72	0.90	92	1.15
13	0.16	33	0.41	53	0.66	73	0.91	93	1.16
14	0.17	34	0.42	54	0.67	74	0.92	94	1.17
15	0.18	35	0.43	55	0.68	75	0.93	95	1.18
16	0.20	36	0.45	56	0.70	76	0.95	96	1.20
17	0.21	37	0.46	57	0.71	77	0.96	97	1.21
18	0.22	38	0.47	58	0.72	78	0.97	98	1.22
19	0.23	39	0.49	59	0.73	79	0.98	99	1.23
20	0.25	40	0.50	60	0.75	80	1.00	100	1.25

EAR INFECTIONS

Infected ears are a common issue for dogs and cats. People often ask what they can do for their pets with ear infections. Ear infections can be prevented if the owner looks at the ear canal. When it appears dirty, either clean the ear (see below) or take the pet to see the pet's doctor. There are so many bugs that can infect the ear that an ear infection is best left to the pet's doctor for treatment. Ear mites are a common problem and often cause ear infections.

The ear canal is not a straight shot to the eardrum; it takes a 90-degree turn and then goes directly to the eardrum. To see into the ear, an instrument called an otoscope is often used. Disposable ear otoscopes are available at a low cost at pharmacies. If there is a bad infection, the ear canal is a common site for accumulation of infectious materials.

Bacterial infections are very common in ears and often require antibiotics in order for the ear to heal. The biggest problem with the advanced ear infections is that owners do not recognize or ignore the ears that are infected until the infection becomes quite bad. This can cause excruciating pain.

Unfortunately, many ears are so badly infected that the pet will not let anyone touch the ear or ears. It is not uncommon to see an ear that is full of pus or exudates; frequently a pungent odor immediately gets one's attention. Often the cause of such an infection is due to the bug called *pseudomonas*. The doctor will have all the necessary tools to properly clean the pet's ears—most often under anesthesia due to the pain associated with the infection. If the ear has an advanced infection, there normally is impacted wax and superficial skin that causes a hard material to be in the ear canal. It requires special tools to remove the mass of materials that often block the ear canal.

Another nasty thing that can occur in the ear is yeast infections. Common yeast for animal ears is the infamous Malassezia. This organism is often found on abdomens, causing black skin, itching, and scratching. One can see the importance of keeping pets ears clean. Flop-eared pets are more prone to ear infections because the ear covers the ear canal and does not let in as much air to help keep it dry and clean.

To determine the kind of bug that is causing the infection may require a culture of the ear for infectious exudates. To determine the best antibiotic, sensitivity tests may be ordered. The problem is that there may be so many different kinds of bugs infecting the ear that it becomes complicated.

TREATMENT

As you learned above, ear infections can be very difficult to treat; at times, they may seem untreatable. It can be a doctor's nightmare. Sometimes a change in the PH of the ear canal may treat the infection. This can be done by mixing one cup of vinegar with two cups of water. It is worth a shot.

Gentian violet can be obtained from feed stores and can be effective. The only problem is that the ears will turn blue until the gentian violet wears off. This treatment is only temporary.

These home treatments may be effective, but they will not harm the pet if they are not effective. You can also look online at 1-800 PetMeds to see if they have a product that you want to use. It may require a prescription from your veterinarian, and you may also obtain a diagnosis and medication from your veterinarian.

PREVENTION

The best prevention is to keep the ears clean and make sure your pet does not have ear mites. If you are using Ivermectin as a heartworm preventive, it will treat the ear mites if present. You can also put about one-fourth to one-half of a milliliter (cc) of Ivermectin into each ear, which will treat the ear mites quickly. If you would like to look into your pet's ears, there are disposable and relatively cheap otoscopes available at drugstores, such as CVS and Walgreens.

USE OF GLUCOSAMINE AND CHONDROITIN SULFATE

I looked extensively for any article that showed that glucosamine and chondroitin were effective, but I could not find any such article.

Plumb's Veterinary Drug Handbook states that there is no study that shows that glucosamine and chondroitin are effective.

The National Institute of Health (NIH) studied 2,000 participants. About 20 percent of the people (+/- 400) in the study stated that they thought they had 25 percent improvement. My question is how can a measurement of 25 percent improvement be evaluated with confidence in any individual? One has to assume that respondent effects were placebo responses and not effects caused by glucosamine and chondroitin sulfate.

I discussed this issue with a physician who specializes in human joints. I told him I had not been able to find an article that supports the fact that glucosamine and chondroitin do anything. His response was that there are no articles that show that glucosamine and chondroitin are effective. It does no good for lost cartilage. When cartilage is gone, there is no way to bring it back. However, he said that many people swear by it. If they take it, there is no harm done, but it does nothing for joints.

I have discussed this with other folks who take this—or someone in their family takes the compound—and they swear they feel better in a few minutes. I have found some formulations of glucosamine and chondroitin that have aspirin added, and the person taking the compound may have some effects due to the small amount of aspirin in the product or they have a placebo effect.

I feel badly for those folks who pay for shots or tablets of glucosamine and chondroitin. The client thinks the compound is going to help their pet, and it actually does nothing. Having seen large dollar amounts attached to a shot of glucosamine and chondroitin, I cannot have a clear conscience using a useless drug. Furthermore, it is an expensive over-the-counter drug—and, in my opinion, a waste of your hard-earned money.

TREATMENT

This discussion has not been about a disease, though it could have been a great treatment for an animal with arthritis or joint disease. However, glucosamine and chondroitin sulfate do no good for animals or people. If you take glucosamine and chondroitin and think the compound is the gift from the universe, go with the treatment since it will not cause any harm. However, do not expect any improvements due to giving glucosamine and chondroitin sulfate.

If your veterinary clinic or hospital says they will use the drug, ask them what effect on the condition of the pet is expected. A single injection may cost eighty dollars or more. If you were to pour tap water on the left front foot, it would be as effective as glucosamine and chondroitin sulfate. This is sad—but true.

DID YOU KNOW?

- Did you know fleas cause anemia?
- Did you know that fleas eat tapeworm eggs?
- Did you know that when pets eat fleas that have tapeworm eggs in them, the pet gets tapeworms?
- Did you know that pets can be born with roundworms?
- Did you know that feeding an all-muscle-meat diet to pets will kill the pet?
- Did you know hookworms can kill pets?
- Did you know that newborn puppies can get hookworms from the milk of the mother?
- Did you know that raccoons visiting neighborhoods at night infest yards with fleas?
- Did you know that pregnant women may cause the fetus to become infected with toxoplasmosis if she cleans cat litter during pregnancy?
- Did you know that mosquitoes have to be infected with larvae at least three days before they can infect pets with heartworms?
- Did you know that raccoons and skunks can use outdoor sandboxes that children play in and leave parasitic eggs that can infect people by migrating to the eyes or brain and cause blindness or brain nerve damage?
- Did you know that cat or dog feces in public sandboxes contaminates the sand and causes under-the-skin infections in people who use the sandbox?

- Did you know that cat or dog feces in public sandboxes contaminates the sand and can cause abdominal infestations of roundworms in people?
- Did you know horse feces can contain tetanus germs that cause tetanus or lockjaw?
- Did you known that horse feces with tetanus germs has caused death in people and pets due to infection of tetanus germs?
- Did you know that public health officials feel that a field that has had horses on it should not be used for playing football for fear of tetanus infections?
- Did you know that using horse manure as a fertilizer has caused people to become infected with tetanus and caused death?
- Did you know that milk pasteurization is to prevent tuberculosis and Q fever?
- Did you know that pasteurization temperature is based on Q fever?
- Did you know that high deer populations mean higher, more frequent numbers of Lyme disease?
- Did you know that pug dogs shipped by air have a greater chance of death in the airplane than other breeds of dogs do?
- Did you know that cats can be so badly infected with tapeworms that they can vomit up tapeworms?
- Did you know that all one has to do to treat fleas is put medication on the back of the neck of the pet?
- Did you know that the most frequent cause of cats squatting without anything happening is due to urinary tract infections?
- Did you know that immunizations prevent diseases?
- Did you know that in the Far East, chiggers carry scrub typhus—and you can get it from a chigger bite?
- Did you know that evaporated milk, such as Carnation, or undiluted evaporated milk can be used to treat constipation and hairballs in cats?
- Did you know that dogs eating raw salmon can get salmon poisoning?

- Did you know that a lot of the Western states have bubonic plague, mostly in rodents, and that cats frequently catch the disease from small rodents?
- Did you know that having your dog spayed before the first heat significantly reduces the chance of the dog having mammary tumors?
- Did you know that ticks carry Rocky Mountain spotted fever?
- Did you know that pets can get Rocky Mountain spotted fever?
- Did you know that you can get Lyme disease from ticks?
- Did you know that it takes a tick twenty-four hours to transmit Lyme disease, and early removal of a tick may reduce the potential for Lyme disease infection?
- Did you know that if you see a red circle on your body you had better see a physician to make sure you have not contracted Lyme disease?
- Did you know that grass awns will drill into pets and cause bad infections?
- Did you know that if a pet eats gunpowder, it may burn a hole in the stomach and kill the pet?
- Did you know that if you have a good wellness program with your pet's doctor, your pet will live longer and have a healthier life?
- Did you know that a pet can have a positive heartworm test and not have heartworm disease?
- Did you know that only female heartworms can be diagnosed by a heartworm blood test—and a dog could be full of male worms that cannot be diagnosed by a blood test?
- Did you know that Ivermectin can be used once per month to prevent heartworms?
- Did you know that several cases of Rift Valley Fever, an African disease, occurred in Florida?
- Did you know that newborn kittens do not get hookworms from nursing?

- Did you know that many internal parasites have a migrating phase in the body on the way to the intestines?
- Did you know that when you treat internal parasites, only those specific worms in the intestines are treated?
- Did you know that because of migrating phases of internal parasites, a repeat dose of worm treatment should occur within three weeks after the first treatment?
- Did you know that fleas eat and poop blood?
- Did you know that fleas lay eggs on the pet, but the eggs are not sticky and can fall onto furniture?
- Did you know the new flea medications kill fleas, flea larvae, and eggs?
- Did you know that—without new flea medications—there are a hundred fleas in the house for every flea on the pet?
- Did you know that flea traps work?
- Did you know that you can find flea traps online by putting "My Flea Trap" in the search engine line and websites will pop up?
- Did you know you can search for www.myfleatrap.com, and the flea trap site will pop up?
- Did you know that you can call (888) 722-3069 to order a flea trap?
- Did you know that this flea trap will catch so many fleas that you have to change the sticky paper?
- Did you know that grapes and raisins can kill dogs?
- Did you know that onions and garlic make dogs and cats very sick and can cause death?
- Did you know that you would not have known any of this if you had not purchased this book?

MOVING

Often pet owners move and take their pets with them or abandon them outside. Leaving a pet to fend for itself in an unfamiliar outdoor world is far from being kind to a former pet.

Leaving pets alone outside is not good for the environment or the poor animal left behind to starve or struggle to survive. It would be much better if an owner would surrender the pet to a shelter, which often finds a home for the pet. Another great option is to leave a pet with a person who is willing to find a new owner for the unwanted pet. Whether left with a new owner, a friend who is committed to finding a new home, or a shelter, it is better than leaving the pet alone outside. The best option is to move the pet with you to the new home.

Moving to a new home may be very stressful for the pet. The new home is a strange environment for the cat or dog. I know of a cat that was so scared upon arrival at a new environment that it hid in a room and did not come out for a month. Food, water, and cat litter were placed in the room with the scared cat; in time, the cat started to explorer the new home and settle in with the family. It just takes time and patience on behalf of the owner for the pet to overcome its fear. There have been owners who believed that the cat had some weird disease and had it killed since it did not come out into the new home.

TREATMENT

The best treatment is to have sympathy for the poor pet and do the right thing by taking the pet with you, finding a new home before you move, having a friend find the animal a new home, or turning the pet in to a shelter. These are all reasonable solutions—and what society would expect of good citizens.

PREVENTION

The numbers of abandoned animals are quite staggering, and many are almost starved to death when found. Many pets are likely to have been run over, poisoned, or been victim of some other tragic event before being found or captured.

PARALYSIS DUE TO TICKS

If your outdoor dog is not acting, walking, or breathing right, you may need to consider tick paralysis. If you notice a wobbly back end, paralysis, or respiratory problems, it could be ticks. These are not specific signs for tick paralysis, however, since other conditions may cause similar signs.

My experience with this disease has been sporadic but very rewarding. When diagnosed, this condition has been resolved within hours after the tick that caused the condition was removed.

If you recognize any of these signs, look for ticks on your pet. The tick or ticks causing the problem may be anywhere on the body. My good fortune has been to find the tick between the shoulder blades in every case I have seen. I would look there first. The ticks can be anywhere on the body—head, ears, toes, footpads, legs, or anus. A good look everywhere on the body is suggested.

Leaving ticks on a dog (normally an *Ixodes* tick) can result in death of the pet that is infected with a toxic tick. Signs normally appear within six days after the tick has attached itself. If ticks are not found right away, relook. Just hang in there until the tick is found. If not found, relook every day or two. It is important that any ticks are found and removed.

TREATMENT

The treatment of choice is to remove the tick or ticks that are found on the body. A tick can potentially cause paralysis. I suggest treating the dog with Advantix II, which kills fleas, flea larvae, eggs, mosquitoes, and ticks. Advantix II is available at pet stores, most military PX or BX facilities, and at 1(800) PetMeds. If all else seems to fail, a tick dip can be used to kill any bugs on the dog. This normally kills all bugs and puts an end to the tick paralysis problem.

PREVENTION

Use of a product that kills ticks prior to going outside with your pet is a good practice to follow. Advantix II is a good product and kills ticks. This will most likely prevent tick paralysis from occurring—even if a tick gets on the dog. If preferred, your dog's doctor will also have products that will repel and kill ticks. The doctor may find that the conditions are caused by something other than ticks.

ANEMIA

Anemia is caused by the loss of blood, and there are all kinds of things that can cause anemia.

In dogs, internal parasites (hookworms, coccidia, or blood parasites), internal bleeding, and other things cause blood loss. Cats have a long list of anemia causes as well, including hookworms, coccidia, and blood parasites (hemobartonellosis and babesiosis), onions, and acetaminophen.

When there is noticeable loss of blood, actions need to be taken to correct the blood loss cause since more blood loss could result in death. To determine anemia, or loss of blood, look at the gums of your pet. The gums should be a nice pink and moist. You can check blood flow by pressing your finger on the gums. You will note that the part under your finger will turn white or very light pink and almost white. Remove your finger, and the color should return to pink almost immediately. If it takes two or three seconds to turn pink—or does not turn back to pink—the pet has anemia. I have checked gums on some animals and found white gums. If the gums are white, the pet is in serious trouble. The cause of the blood loss needs to be determined and treated—or the pet could die.

A blood transfusion might be in order to treat the anemia. It does no good to have a blood transfusion if the cause of anemia is not eliminated because the anemia will come charging right back. If the anemia is such that it is a life-or-death issue, a blood transfusion has to be given and the cause of the blood loss must be determined.

Different areas of the country have different common blood-loss causes. In many areas, the most common cause of anemia in dogs and cats is hookworms. I have been in areas of the country where autoimmune-mediated anemia was a common cause. As I have not been in every area of the country, there may be other frequent causes of anemia. Even if hookworms are a common cause of anemia in some areas of the country does not mean that is so where you live.

Hookworm infestations that are bad enough to cause anemia will normally have other recognizable signs. Bloody diarrhea at our facility in Florida is usually caused by hookworms. Hookworms eat blood.

An infestation of many hookworms is a cause of severe anemia. A pet can be alive today and dead tomorrow due to hookworm infestation. One can treat for hookworms. However, it is always best to have a fecal sample run to determine that hookworms are causing the loose stools. There is always a chance that bloody diarrhea is caused by coccidia, which is a protozoan parasite that causes the same signs as hookworms. Coccidia in our area are rare. In other areas, it might be the main cause of loose stools. Fecal exams will ensure that you are treating the correct parasite.

Fleas can be a cause of rather severe anemia as well. This is due to the animal not being treated for fleas. I have seen flea infections so bad that the hair on the dog was coated with blood and looked like red taffy had been poured on the body. The hairs clicked and cracked when touched due to the amount of blood on the hair. It was bad. In our facility, it is not uncommon to find anemic dogs that have been badly infested with fleas.

TREATMENT

As you have learned, many things cause blood loss, and it may be quite difficult to determine the cause of the anemia. However, if you are a diehard, do-it-yourself dude, you can treat for hookworms with Panacur (Fenbendazole). The dosage chart by body weight can be found in the chart below (Table 2.4). Look for your pet's weight to obtain the proper dosage. You can purchase Panacur or Fenbendazole at Petco, PetSmart, and 1 (800) PetMeds. If you purchase from the pet stores or 1 (800) PetMeds, follow the directions on the package the drug comes in. If you purchase Panacur at the feed store, make sure you purchase 100 mg/cc to enable you to use Table 2.4. You can also treat for coccidia using Tables 2.5 and 2.6. Tables 2.5 and 2.6 are based on the product available at feed stores, which is called Sulmet 12.5 percent solution. Sulmet (Sulfadimethoxine) is a liquid that comes in a rather large container. The volume is far more than you will ever need.

Sulmet is labeled for use with chickens. It is the same compound

Sulfadimethoxine, which is used to treat coccidia in pets. 1 (800) PetMeds has a product called Albon (Sulfadimethoxine) in tablet form. It takes a prescription to purchase Albon. You can purchase by the tablet, but you must purchase a minimum number of tablets. Due to costs and the large volumes you will obtain, I feel it is much better to have your pet's doctor diagnose coccidia and let the doctor provide the medications. This is much easier, a lot more convenient, and may be cheaper.

PREVENTION

If you are using Ivermectin to prevent heartworms, you will also be treating hookworms, roundworms, and whipworms at the same time. In cats, Ivermectin will prevent heartworms and treat hookworms and roundworms. If you use Revolution flea medication, you will also treat internal parasites. Ivermectin is available at feed stores, but you will need a prescription for Revolution. With a prescription, you can obtain Revolution from 1-800 PetMeds. If your veterinarian sells it, you can purchase it from your veterinarian.

Table 2.4 Panacur (Fenbendazole) Dose-by-Weight Chart

100 mg/cc Panacur [Fenbendazole] Dosing Chart
Repeat the dose for three days and then repeat
the three-day treatment in two weeks.
(weight times 25 divided by 100 = dose in cc)

Weight Pounds	Dose cc	Weight Pounds	Dose cc	Weight Pounds	Dose cc	Weight Pounds	Dose cc	Weight Pounds	Dose cc
1	0.25	21	5.25	41	10.25	61	15.25	81	20.25
2	0.50	22	5.50	42	10.50	62	15.50	82	20.50
3	0.75	23	5.75	43	10.75	63	15.75	83	20.75
4	1.0	24	6.0	44	11.00	64	16.0	84	21.0
5	1.25	25	6.25	45	11.25	65	16.25	85	21.25
6	1.50	26	6.50	46	11.50	66	16.50	86	21.50
7	1.75	27	6.75	47	11.75	67	16.75	87	21.75
8	2.0	28	7.0	48	12.0	68	17.0	88	22.0
9	2.25	29	7.25	49	12.25	69	17.25	89	22.25
10	2.50	30	7.50	50	12.50	70	17.50	90	22.50
11	2.75	31	7.75	51	12.75	71	17.75	91	22.75
12	3.00	32	8.0	52	13.0	72	18.0	92	23.0
13	3.25	33	8.25	53	13.25	73	18.25	93	23.25
14	3.50	34	8.50	54	13.50	74	18.50	94	23.50
15	3.75	35	8.75	55	13.75	75	18.75	95	23.75
16	4.00	36	9.0	56	14.0	76	19.0	96	24.0
17	4.25	37	9.25	57	14.25	77	19.25	97	24.25
18	4.50	38	9.50	58	14.50	78	19.50	98	24.50
19	4.75	39	9.75	59	14.75	79	19.75	99	24.75
20	5.00	40	10.0	60	15.0	80	20.0	100	25.0

Table 2.5 Dog and Cat Day 1 Sulmet (Sulfadimethoxine) Dose-by-Weight Chart

12.5 Percent Sulmet (Sulfadimethoxine 125 mg/cc)
(weight divided by 5 = dose in cc)
Administer by mouth only.
If desired, dilute with water and double the volume.

Weight Pounds	Dose cc	Weight Pounds	Dose cc	Weight Pounds	Dose cc	Weight Pounds	Dose cc	Weight Pounds	Dose cc
1	0.2	21	4.2	41	8.2	61	12.2	81	16.2
2	0.4	22	4.4	42	8.4	62	12.4	82	16.4
3	0.6	23	4.6	43	8.6	63	12.6	83	16.6
4	0.8	24	4.8	44	8.8	64	12.8	84	16.8
5	1.0	25	5.0	45	9.0	65	13.0	85	17.0
6	1.2	26	5.2	46	9.2	66	13.2	86	17.2
7	1.4	27	5.4	47	9.4	67	13.4	87	17.4
8	1.6	28	5.6	48	9.6	68	13.6	88	17.6
9	1.8	29	5.8	49	9.8	69	13.8	89	17.8
10	2.0	30	6.0	50	10	70	14.0	90	18.0
11	2.2	31	6.2	51	10.2	71	14.2	91	18.2
12	2.4	32	6.4	52	10.4	72	14.4	92	18.4
13	2.6	33	6.6	53	10.6	73	14.6	93	18.6
14	2.8	34	6.8	54	10.8	74	14.8	94	18.8
15	3.0	35	7.0	55	11.0	75	15.0	95	19.0
16	3.2	36	7.2	56	11.2	76	15.2	96	19.2
17	3.4	37	7.4	57	11.4	77	15.4	97	19.4
18	3.6	38	7.6	58	11.6	78	15.6	98	19.6
19	3.8	39	7.8	59	11.8	79	15.8	99	19.8
20	4.0	40	8.0	60	12.0	80	16.0	100	2.0

Table 2.6 Dog and Cat Days 2–5 Sulmet (Sulfadimethoxine) Dose-by-Weight Chart

12.5 Percent Sulmet (Sulfadimethoxine 125 mg/cc)
(divide day one dose by 2 = dose in cc)
Administer by mouth only.
If desired, dilute with water and double the volume.

Weight Pounds	Dose cc	Weight Pounds	Dose cc	Weight Pounds	Dose cc	Weight Pounds	Dose cc	Weight Pounds	Dose cc
1	0.1	21	2.1	41	4.1	61	6.1	81	8.1
2	0.2	22	2.2	42	4.2	62	6.2	82	8.2
3	0.3	23	2.3	43	4.3	63	6.3	83	8.3
4	0.4	24	2.4	44	4.4	64	6.4	84	8.4
5	0.5	25	2.5	45	4.5	65	6.5	85	8.5
6	0.6	26	2.6	46	4.6	66	6.6	86	8.6
7	0.7	27	2.7	47	4.7	67	6.7	87	8.7
8	0.8	28	2.8	48	4.8	68	6.8	88	8.8
9	0.9	29	2.9	49	4.9	69	6.9	89	8.9
10	1.0	30	3.0	50	5.0	70	7.0	90	9.0
11	1.1	31	3.1	51	5.1	71	7.1	91	9.1
12	1.2	32	3.2	52	5.2	72	7.2	92	9.2
13	1.3	33	3.3	53	5.3	73	7.3	93	9.3
14	1.4	34	3.4	54	5.4	74	7.4	94	9.4
15	1.5	35	3.5	55	5.5	75	7.5	95	9.5
16	1.6	36	3.6	56	5.6	76	7.6	96	9.6
17	1.7	37	3.7	57	5.7	77	7.7	97	9.7
18	1.8	38	3.8	58	5.8	78	7.8	98	9.8
19	1.9	39	3.9	59	5.9	79	7.9	99	9.9
20	2.0	40	4.0	60	6.0	80	8.0	100	10.0

PERSISTENT LOOSE STOOLS (DIARRHEA)

We have seen many a dog or cat that has had persistent loose stools or diarrhea. It is an exasperating experience—and often is an issue that pet owners will not tolerate for any length of time.

An easy diet of cottage cheese and cooked rice seems to be the pixie dust to rescue the pet from this kind of problem. This diet comes from my residency at the University of California–Davis—thanks to my mentor Dr. Donald Strombeck. While I was a resident there, several pets were referred to the teaching hospital with persistent diarrhea. This diet provided a quick solution to loose stools. I came away thinking if I learned nothing else, this was the one thing to know—and it seems to work all the time for cats and dogs. I was completely surprised that cats would consume this homemade diet, but they seem to do so.

Many things will cause loose stools—viruses, bacteria overloads, internal parasites, and food allergies. There is a grocery list of other causes. This diet tends to solve the loose-stool problems. There is not one product that is 100 percent effective. I have yet to have a case of persistent loose stools that this diet did not help, but your pet could be a first.

Follow the diet for at least two weeks before evaluating the effectiveness of the diet as a control for loose stools. It is important that no other foods be fed or be available to the pet. This includes table scraps. If this protocol is not followed, you cannot expect the cottage-cheese-and-rice diet to be effective. Pets have been fed this diet for months with no issues. When normal stools are being passed again, you can return to the normal diet. If the normal diet seems to be the cause, restart the cottage-cheese-and-rice diet—and consult with your pet's doctor for your next move. A diet of cottage cheese and rice using these amounts of cottage cheese and rice will provide 820 Kcal:

Use an eight-fluid-ounce cup for measuring. Add two volumes of water to seven ounces of rice and cook. When cooked, add three and one-half to four ounces of cottage cheese. This produces a diet of 22–25 percent cottage cheese and 18–20 percent of protein on a dry matter basis.

I have found that most people will not follow the above because they do not want to make such a small amount. Follow these directions for mixing the cottage cheese and rice.

Table 2.7 Rice-and-Cottage-Cheese Diarrhea Diet

- Use one cup of *instant rice* to four ounces of cottage cheese.
- Fix four cups of *instant rice*. Cool the rice in the refrigerator. After the rice is cool, mix sixteen ounces of cottage cheese with the rice (you can purchase cottage cheese in sixteen-ounce or one-pound containers).
- Feed the rice and cottage cheese to the dog or cat. The rice and cottage cheese not being fed should be kept in the refrigerator until it is used.
- Do not feed any other food with this diet.

MY CAT EATS A LOT BUT IS LOSING WEIGHT

This discussion is for the benefit of those who have a cat that eats a lot of food but seems to keep losing weight. There are several causes, but the two most common causes are the overproduction of thyroid hormone by the thyroid gland and diabetes mellitus. Diabetes is the result of a lack of insulin production by the pancreas. These conditions are most often referred to as hyperthyroidism and diabetes respectfully.

Some other less common causes of overeating and weight loss include chronic internal parasites, maldigestion syndrome, malabsorption syndromes, poor quality of foods being fed, and the pancreas not properly secreting digestive enzymes into the intestinal tract. There are other devastating diseases like cancer that cause similar signs as those mentioned with this discussion.

Some signs that might be seen with the overproduction of thyroid hormones include intermittent vomiting and diarrhea; diabetes signs may be abnormal amounts of water consumption and excessive urination. These signs are somewhat subtle signs and may not be recognized by you as a problem until there is excessive weight loss in the pet.

It has to be remembered that these conditions do not happen overnight. They develop slowly over time. The main weight-loss causes are more commonly noted in cats that are seven years of age and older. That does not mean that other ages are exempt since it can happen to cats of any age. In advanced stages of these conditions, a cat may show the most common signs of excessive water consumption and urination.

TREATMENT

It is obvious that diagnosis and treatment medications will need to be determined by the pet's doctor. Both primary and less common causes need to be properly diagnosed and appropriate medications dispensed at befitting dosages—and require days or months of treatment.

PREVENTION

The two most common causes are insidious and difficult to prevent. However, keeping a cat's weight within proper weight ranges and not overfeeding will help prevent diabetes. This is another reason to have a preventive medicine program for your pet. These conditions can be diagnosed early and may limit or even prevent the disease from affecting your pet.

COLLECTING FECAL SAMPLES

Collection of fecal samples is a rather simple task, and it is important that the fecal sample is fresh to ensure a correct diagnosis. First of all, it does not take pounds for a sample. A few grams are sufficient for a proper fecal sample. It is best to collect immediately after the pet voids to ensure that a fresh and correct sample will be examined. This will ensure that the sample collected is not vomitus or some other medical sample that will not provide a correct diagnosis.

Fresh samples are important since time and temperature allow for changes of any parasite egg and may cause an incorrect identification of the parasite. In addition, some free-living bugs may invade the sample and hatch, causing confusion with identification with some lungworms. The reason you spend time and effort to collect the sample in the first place is to find out if there is indeed a parasite present; if you identity the parasite correctly, it can be treated with the proper drugs.

If it is not possible to quickly get the fecal sample to the correct location for examination within an hour or two, the sample should be refrigerated. Do not freeze the sample because the freezing can distort some parasite identification parameters. If there is reason to believe your pet is infested with giardia or trichomonads, the sample should be evaluated within thirty minutes of collection to ensure that the parasite can even be seen in the test. These parasites are destroyed quickly, permitting a misdiagnosis of the parasite due to it not being present in the test sample.

TREATMENT

Many parasites can be treated with the same drugs, but some require special medications. Parasites can be a health hazard to people as well as pets, and it is important that a good exam is completed. Most intestinal parasites can be treated with Panacur using the following dosage chart (Table 2.8). Look up the weight of the pet and get the number of cc you need to treat the pet.

Panacur 100 mg per milliliter or cc is available at feed stores. You can also purchase this product at PetSmart, 1 (800) PetMeds, or Petco. If you do this, follow the directions on the package. Panacur will treat hookworms, roundworms, whipworms, tapeworms, and giardia parasites.

PREVENTION

Routine treatment keeps parasites under control. A fecal exam every six or twelve months is good plan for your pet. If multiple negatives are noted, extending fecal exams to every two years is reasonable.

However, some pets manage to become reinfected more often than others do.

Table 2.8 *Panacur (Fenbendazole) Dose-by-Weight Chart*

100 mg/cc Panacur [Fenbendazole] Dosing Chart
Repeat the dose for three days and then repeat
the three-day treatment in two weeks.
(weight times 25 divided by 100 = dose in cc)

Weight Pounds	Dose cc	Weight Pounds	Dose cc	Weight Pounds	Dose cc	Weight Pounds	Dose cc	Weight Pounds	Dose cc
1	0.25	21	5.25	41	10.25	61	15.25	81	20.25
2	0.50	22	5.50	42	10.50	62	15.50	82	20.50
3	0.75	23	5.75	43	10.75	63	15.75	83	20.75
4	1.0	24	6.0	44	11.00	64	16.0	84	21.0
5	1.25	25	6.25	45	11.25	65	16.25	85	21.25
6	1.50	26	6.50	46	11.50	66	16.50	86	21.50
7	1.75	27	6.75	47	11.75	67	16.75	87	21.75
8	2.0	28	7.0	48	12.0	68	17.0	88	22.0
9	2.25	29	7.25	49	12.25	69	17.25	89	22.25
10	2.50	30	7.50	50	12.50	70	17.50	90	22.50
11	2.75	31	7.75	51	12.75	71	17.75	91	22.75
12	3.00	32	8.0	52	13.0	72	18.0	92	23.0
13	3.25	33	8.25	53	13.25	73	18.25	93	23.25
14	3.50	34	8.50	54	13.50	74	18.50	94	23.50
15	3.75	35	8.75	55	13.75	75	18.75	95	23.75
16	4.00	36	9.0	56	14.0	76	19.0	96	24.0
17	4.25	37	9.25	57	14.25	77	19.25	97	24.25
18	4.50	38	9.50	58	14.50	78	19.50	98	24.50
19	4.75	39	9.75	59	14.75	79	19.75	99	24.75
20	5.00	40	10.0	60	15.0	80	20.0	100	25.0

HEAD TILT

Infections of the ear may be the most common cause of head tilt. Head tilt can also be due to central brain disorders. Tilt of the head is seen when the head leans to the left or to the right. The infection, if present, is in the inner ear and affects the balance mechanisms of the inner ear.

A pet's doctor calls this the vestibular system. If the head tilt is due to infection, the infection will be on the side of the head tilt.

The differential between head tilt and head turn needs to be determined by the pet's doctor. A head turn is turning the head to one side, which is a brain issue. If both ears happen to have an infection at the same time, there may not be any signs of head tilt. There may be a back-and-forth movement of the eye. There may also be a slow moment in one direction and a fast movement in the opposite direction. The eye movement may be more noticeable if you elevate the head. There may be some facial nerve issues or noticeable dry eye on the side of the tilt.

TREATMENT
It is my belief that this is an issue for the pet's doctor to properly diagnose and treat.

PREVENTION
Here is where you can shine. It is simple to keep ears clean and free from ear mites. This will prevent inner ear infections. In addition to your efforts, your preventive medicine program will be one of the benefits obtained by having the program. The ears will be checked at each physical during the preventive medicine checkups.

LYME DISEASE

Lyme disease is one of the most common tick-transmitted zoonotic diseases in the world. Where there are an increased numbers of ticks, deer, and mice, there is an increased number of Lyme disease–infected animals and people. This disease is caused by spirochete bacteria called *Borrela burgdorferi*. In dogs, it causes a dominant clinical sign for recurrent lameness and depression. Dogs may develop kidney disease, neurologic signs, or heart conditions.

After dogs are attacked by a tick, a generalized infection of connective tissue in joints, tendons, muscles, and lymph nodes most often occurs within a week or a month. These signs are a basis for the thought that Lyme disease might be the cause of lameness in dogs. The signs are not necessarily a flashing light to identify Lyme disease, but they certainly make one think of Lyme disease as a culprit. This is especially true in certain areas within the United States; 90 percent of all Lyme disease cases occur in in New England. Lyme disease cases also occur in the northern Midwest, California, and some Southern states.

Signs of possible Lyme-disease infection in your pet might include recurrent lameness, an acute form of lameness that lasts for three to four days, swollen joints, and pain when pressure is applied by squeezing the joint areas. The good news is that if you do not ignore these signs, antibiotics will work well at this point. If the signs are ignored, this can develop into several joints becoming a nonerosive arthritic joint. Your pet may walk with a stiff gait and have an arched back. Superficial lymph nodes close to the tick bite may be swollen. Heart involvement is rare, but it can include a complete heart blockage. Neurologic complications are rare. That does not rule out the possibility of a neurologic sign.

Ticks are the bad guys with the symbolic black hats when it comes to Lyme disease. These dudes live about two years. The new larvae hatch in the spring and become infected with the Lyme disease bacteria *Borrela burgdorferi* when they feed on small mammals. The most common rodent providing meals for the ticks is the white-footed mouse. The adult ticks like to feed on larger animals, such as deer. After finishing a meal on the deer, the adult tick drops off and hides under leaves until spring—and then lays about two thousand eggs. Male ticks do not attach and do not have a blood meal like the females do.

Lyme disease is an excellent example of how diseases can spread over the country in short periods of time. At one time, this disease was found mostly New England. New England, not wanting to be selfish, shared it with the rest of the country. This and other diseases are spread by transient populations and the quick, long-distance transportation now available in the world.

TREATMENT

This disease is one for your pet's doctor to accurately diagnose and properly treat.

PREVENTION

Whenever your pet goes into an area that might have ticks, it is important the dog receives a good going-over to find ticks on its body. Using Advantix or Activyl flea medications that also repel or kill ticks is a good plan to follow. Another good plan is to dip the dog after each outing to kill any bugs that may have gotten on your dog—especially if the area your pet has been in is known to have ticks.

BLOOD IN FECES

There are two kinds of blood found in feces of pets. The black blood is due to digestion of blood, normally coming from high in the intestinal tract. This kind of blood makes the feces look black. The other type of blood comes from low in the digestive tract, and this blood is red. If either is seen, one needs to find the cause since neither is normal for dogs or cats.

There can be many causes of the dark blood feces or bleeding high in the intestinal tract. It may be due to issues in the intestines. Cancer can be the cause and may have invaded the intestines.

Some causes of black feces or "melena" include benign polyps, infectious causes, foreign bodies, infections, cancers, inability to clot blood, and nonsteroid anti-inflammatory drugs. Even ingestion of raw meats can be a cause, and many others are not listed.

TREATMENT

This is an important issue that needs the expertise of your pet's doctor as soon as dark black feces due to bleeding or fresh red blood are noted.

PREVENTION

This is an issue that emphasizes the need for a wellness program since this is one of the things that most likely will be prevented. If Pepto-Bismol is being used, this will make the stools look black.

HEATSTROKE

Heatstroke is not an unusual occurrence in areas of the country with temperatures above 90° F (32.2° C). When it is hot outside and pet dogs are in the outdoors, it is not uncommon for them to be panting and have body temperatures of 103° F (39.4° C). This temperature is above normal 102° F (38.8° C), but it is quite common—and is not considered to be an abnormal temperature when the environmental temperatures are high. Body temperatures can be elevated by infections or caused by the environment. This discussion will focus on the environmental heat that causes heatstroke in dogs and cats. Cats seldom experience heatstroke, but they are affected by the heat; they pant and do not do well. Cats appear to be sick until their body temperatures return to about 102° F (38.8° C).

To start this discussion, let's set the stage for understanding how the body works when it is exposed to elevated temperatures or low temperatures. Think of the skin of the body as a radiator just like the one in your car. The purpose of the car radiator is to transfer heat and provide a cooling system for your car. The skin of the body works very similar to a car radiator. When it is hot, the body mechanism works to expel the heat. When it is cold, the body works to conserve heat. Have you ever washed dishes in hot water and noticed that your forehead starts to sweat? Heat is being transferred from the hands to the internal body temperature. The body, head, foot, and hands are all a part of the heat-exchange system and gain heat or lose heat according to the outside temperatures. These body parts are important in the heat-exchange system of the body. When it is hot, blood vessels carry more blood to the skin to exchange more heat. When it is cold, the skin blood vessels contract or carry less blood so the blood can pool in the central body to allow for conservation of heat.

In summer months with elevated temperatures, a dog will pant and let its tongue hang out of its mouth. This is for the purpose of losing heat. Dogs do not sweat, which contributes to making the dog's skin a poor heat exchanger. The dog builds up body temperature faster in hot environments than other animals with better heat-exchanging skin. People and horses sweat and lose body heat in that way. In hot weather, dogs can get elevated temperatures in very short periods of time.

In Florida, it is not unusual to have temperatures above 90° F (32.2° C) in the summer. The following examples are actual events that occurred in hot weather. A man and his black-haired dog walked a mile in the heat of the day on a blacktop road to the grocery store. They walked home, but the dog collapsed a short distance from their home. The temperature of the dog was so high that it would not register on the thermometer.

In another incident, an animal-control officer noticed a person on a bicycle with his dog running beside the bicycle in the heat of the day. As he looked at the dog, it collapsed on the road and died. The body temperature of the second dog is not known, but the temperature was high enough to kill it.

The critical temperature in pets that leads to organ damage or dysfunction is about 109° F (42.7° C). The organs involved are the kidneys, the brain, the heart, and others. Humidity adds to the likelihood of heatstroke. Signs of impending heatstroke include humidity, panting, tongue hanging out, elevated temperature, hyper-salivation, and very dark red gums in the mouth. Very red gums are an easy thing to look for.

My friend walked his Doberman over the top of a dam on a gravel road. He said the dog looked exhausted. He noted the tongue looked fiery red. He and his dog were by a lake. The dog walked into the lake and stayed until the mucous membranes of the mouth returned to normal before heading home.

TREATMENT

When treating a dog for heat stroke, it is important to remember that the skin is like a radiator. When the skin is hot, the blood vessels carry more blood to the surface for cooling. When cold, the blood vessels contract and conserve heat. If you put ice on your dog's skin, the blood vessels will contract and start to conserve heat—the opposite of what you are trying to do. It's important to run cool water over the dog. Normal running water, if not heated by the heat of the day, is best for the dog. The sooner the signs of heatstroke are recognized and the treatment is started, the better the chances for the dog. *Early recognition is the key to successful treatment of heatstroke.*

PREVENTION

Do not exercise or walk the dog in very hot weather. Wait for a cooler part of the day for quality dog time. On very hot days, it is still quite hot in shady areas. Unfortunately, it is easy to lose a dog to heatstroke in very hot weather. Be wise—not sad.

NASAL DISCHARGE

Nasal discharge is a common issue in multiple kennel operations and is most often due to an infection caused by bacteria or a virus. There are other causes, but the most common are mild nasal infections. Other signs associated with this problem include lung infections, discharge associated with swallowing, or cleft palates. Some eye infections produce excessive tears and will drain by the nasal-eye duct, causing watery discharge from the nose. Foreign bodies in the nose and tumors may be other causes.

The challenge with nasal discharge is determining the cause and treating it. If a foreign body is causing the discharge, the removal of the foreign body will stop the discharge. If it is an eye that is producing excess tears, treating the eye will resolve the nasal discharge. If it happens to be an infectious process, antibiotics will resolve the nasal discharge.

Do not confuse a nasal discharge with a fresh lick of the nose. This can be misleading. Normally an owner will be familiar with the healthy look of his or her pet and will be able to identify abnormal nasal discharge.

Early recognition of the discharge may lead to the proper steps to correct the condition rapidly—and is the best approach for this condition. Normally, delays in seeking help or correcting the nasal discharge yourself can result in difficult resolution of the issue.

TREATMENT

It is not rocket science, but the cause of the nasal discharge has to be identified before any treatment can occur. As an owner, you can look in the nose. If there happens to be a stick inside one of the nasal passages, you can pull it out. If you cannot identify a cause, you will need the assistance of your pet's doctor.

PREVENTION

There is little a person can do since no one has a crystal ball to determine what will happen in the future. However, if you are a hunter and your pet's nose starts to run, look for foreign bodies. It happens more often than you can imagine.

MAMMARY GLAND INFECTION (MASTITIS)

Mammary gland infections seem to come in three packages. The first is due to some sort of trauma that allows for infection on the skin, including the mammary glands. Early withdrawal of the young from the mother allows excessive milk to accumulate in the mammary glands and allows bacterial infections to occur. The first scenario for the early withdrawal for feeding young is that the dog ends up in a shelter—and no one shows up to claim the pet. The second early withdrawal is that the owner gives the puppies away too early—and the mammary glands are full of unused milk that causes infections to occur. On occasion, a mammary gland infection may occur from an unknown source during nursing.

Mammary infections need attention—or the pet will become very ill. Signs in a postdelivery pet with a mammary gland infection include not eating, lethargy, or neglecting the young. The newborns will not be healthy, will lose weight, and may die. The mammary glands normally become large and feel hot and firm when palpated. They are often distended due to engorged retention of milk.

TREATMENT

Whenever there is enlargement of the mammary, the pet needs to see the pet's doctor to start antibiotics or determine that the pet is okay. Postponement in treating mammary gland infections often results in rupture and discharge of exudates.

PREVENTION

Keeping the pet clean and healthy is the best thing to do. A preventive medicine program is a great idea for an expectant dog or cat.

ANAPHYLAXIS

Anaphylaxis is a severe reaction to a bee or wasp sting or a drug that stimulates a reaction in the body to cause difficulty breathing, hives, edema, skin swelling, pale gums, shock, and possible death. People with severe reactions to bee stings need medication to reverse the reaction. This occurs in pets as well. Frequently it is has a very rapid onset.

The cause of death is often due to the effects that this type of reaction has on the heart. This type of reaction can occur when immunizations are given to pets as well. Perhaps you have had a personal immunization and have been asked to wait before leaving due to what could be a reaction to the immunization in your body. So it is with pets. Anaphylaxis can occur in any dog or cat, and there is no species, age, or sex predilection. One and all can be involved.

There are some dogs that seem to be more prone to an anaphylactic response. Pit bulls and boxers are the most frequently affected with urticaria. Urticaria is a hypersensitivity that causes red skin lesions and a scratching sensation.

The trigger for this type of reaction can be stings from bees, wasps, fire ants, or other insects, food, immunizations, surgeries, blood loss, trauma, antibiotics, parasite treatment medications, and snakebites. There are many other stimulators that cause anaphylaxis.

An event can cause a second exposure to be much more severe. The problem is that the first event may not have been recognized or noted. The second event may seem like the first occurrence, but it may be a later response to those that may have set the stage for a whopper of a reaction that can cause death.

Signs to look for include red spots forming on the skin, which may be large or small, weakness, depression, vomiting, uncontrolled defecating or urination, pale gums which become less pink or turn white or very pale, and coma. In addition, cats may show difficulty in respiration or collapse. If it occurs due to an insect, the stinger may be found. If a stinger is found, look for a small bulb on the end. The end in the skin has a barb like a fish hook; if one squeezes the bulb to remove the stinger, more venom will be injected into the skin of the pet. So be careful removing any stingers.

TREATMENT

Mild reactions can be treated with Benadryl, which is diphenhydramine HCL to be given at 4.4 mg/lbs. or 2 mg/kg two times daily. For severe reactions, medical help may be necessary, and delay in getting professional help may result in death. In small dogs, it is not uncommon to have mild reactions to immunizations—weakness, pale gums, inability to get up, or unwillingness to walk. Some will have loose stools and urinate. If one has children's Benadryl, three to five milliliters or cubic centimeters can be given by mouth. Recovery will normally take about fifteen or twenty minutes.

PREVENTION

It is impossible to know when a pet may have a reaction until it happens. If you have a pet that has had reactions, premedication before immunization may be of benefit for the pet. Tell your veterinarian about any reactions the pet may have had. This is one item that lots of people will lie about to their veterinarians, and it may be responsible for the death of a pet. *Please do not lie to your veterinarian.*

Table 2.9 *Benadryl Dog and Cat Dose-by-Weight Chart*

Benadryl for Dogs and Cats Target Dose of 2 Mg/Lbs.

25 mg tablets are available OTC. Dosage is based on cut
25 mg tablets, which cannot be precisely accurate.
Remember dose is close—not accurate due to cut tablets.

Weight Pounds	Dose # Tablets and/or Tablet Parts	Weight Pounds	Dose # Tablets and/or Tablet Parts	Weight Pounds	Dose # Tablets and/or Tablet Parts	Weight Pounds	Dose # Tablets and/or Tablet Parts	Weight Pounds	Dose # Tablets and/or Tablet Parts
1	1/8=.12	21	1.75	41	3.25	61	5	81	6.50
2	¼= .25	22	1.75	42	3.25	62	5	82	6.50
3	¼=.25	23	1.75	43	3.50	63	5	83	6.75
4	½+¼ =3/4 =.75	24	2	44	3.50	64	5.12	84	6.75
5	½=.50	25	2	45	3.75	65	5.25	85	6.75
6	½=.50	26	2	46	3.75	66	5.25	86	6
7	½=.50	27	2.12	47	3.75	67	5.25	87	6.75+.12
8	.50+.12	28	2.25	48	3.75	68	5.50	88	7
9	.50+.25	29	2.25	49	3.75+.12	69	5.50	89	7
10	.50+.25	30	2.50	50	4	70	5.50	90	7.25
11	1	31	2.50	51	4	71	5.75	91	7.25
12	1	32	2.50	52	4.12	72	5.75	92	7.25
13	1	33	2.75	53	4.25	73	5.75	93	7.50
14	1.12	34	2.75	54	4.25	74	6	94	7.50
15	1.25	35	2.75	55	4.50	75	6	95	7.50
16	1.25	36	2.75+.12	56	4.50	76	6	96	7.75
17	1.25	37	3	57	4.50	77	6.12	97	7.75
18	1.50	38	3	58	4.50	78	6.25	98	8
19	1.50	39	3.12	59	4.75	79	6.25	99	8
20	1.50+.12	40	3.25	60	4.75	80	6.50	100	8

1/8 = .12 tablet, ¼ = .25 tablet, ½ = .5 tablet, ½ + ¼ = ¾ = .75 tab

VACCINATIONS OF DOGS AND CATS

It is always best to take your pet to see your pet's doctor for vaccinations. However, if you're a do-it-yourself person, here are some guidelines for you to follow as you immunize your pets. It is very important that pets receive vaccines. It makes no sense to have pets and allow them to get sick with diseases that can kill when those diseases can be prevent by simple vaccinations. Almost all vaccines for pets can be purchased at a feed store (with the exception of rabies vaccines).

When giving vaccines, you need to be aware that some animals do nothing when the needle is inserted under the skin. Others attempt to bite—so it is a good idea to prepare and be cautious when vaccinating. If you have vaccinated your pets before, you already know how they normally react, but one never knows from one time to the next. You should take the appropriate steps to prevent biting or scratching when doing any procedure on your pet.

You need to wash your wounds if bitten or scratched, and you may need to see your physician if it is a bad wound or more than a simple scratch. Wounds can become infected and can require lots of medical attention. You might think this is common sense, but experience has shown it not to be so. Therefore, be wise and do not be hospitalized because you did not think it was important. Believe me, it has happened. Do not let it happen to you. Just prepare and take steps so your pet will not bite or scratch you or your helper.

Some vaccines given to pets can cause reactions. Most are minor, but you need to be aware and watch for possible life-threating reactions. Almost all reactions occur in small breeds of dogs. You might recall that when you received your last vaccination in your arm the nurse made you hang around for fifteen or twenty minutes. This is to make sure that you did not have a reaction to the vaccine. Furthermore, if your pet has had reactions to vaccines in the past, *do not vaccinate* them. Take them to the pet's doctor for the safety of the pet. My experience with vaccination reactions is that most reactions occur within twenty minutes after giving the vaccine, but some can take longer. Almost all reactions occur in small breeds of dogs.

A normal response to diphenhydramine (Benadryl) is good. You must have this over-the-counter drug on hand when you are giving vaccinations. It will not do much good if you have to run to a store to get diphenhydramine. Many people panic when their pet has a reaction to vaccines. If you're one that becomes panicky, I suggest that you not vaccinate your pets. You need to be able to function to treat your pet. I know it sounds silly, but it has often been observed at immunization clinics. The following are some minor signs that may occur. We hope you never see any of them, but it is best to be prepared. You need to be able to recognize them if they occur. We hope you never have a need to treat a vaccine reaction, but it does happen.

- discomfort and possible swelling at the vaccination site
- mild fever
- decreased appetite and activity
- sneezing, mild coughing, runny nose, or minor respiratory changes
- pale gums

The following are more-serious and perhaps less-common signs:

- vomiting and/or diarrhea
- itchy skin may seem bumpy (possible hives)
- swelling of the muzzle and around the face, neck, or eyes
- severe coughing or difficulty breathing
- lying down and not getting up
- pale gums
- collapsing

TREATMENT

Small dogs can be treated with children's liquid Benadryl, which has 12.5 mg in 5 ml. This is normally sufficient for minor reactions, and a dose of 1.5 to 2 mg per pound or 2 to 4 mg/kg of body weight is a good dose.

Time is on your side since most minor reactions will resolve without medication within thirty minutes. However, the diphenhydramine will hasten the recovery. When they start walking and wagging their tails, they are normally okay. Diphenhydramine (Benadryl) can be purchased at grocery stores, Walmart, pharmacies, and military PX and BX facilities. These stores also have 1 and 2 mg tablets that may be easier to use than the liquid. If you feel uncomfortable giving vaccines, go to the pet's doctor. Do not hesitate—just go. If you see a severe reaction, it is necessary to go directly to your pet's doctor. Do not attempt to treat your pet for severe reactions.

NECESSARY VACCINATIONS

Vaccinations have progressed a long way in the past forty years. Vaccinations for animals are now broken down into two groups, and they are designated as core or noncore vaccinations. Essentially pet needs are limited to core vaccines unless there are unusual circumstances, special requirements, or needs. Noncore vaccines are recommended only when needed.

Bordetella is a good example of a required vaccine for boarding of animals. Another example might be an outbreak of a disease that can be prevented by a noncore vaccine or some other need as determined for a specific area. The good news is that you may not need a bunch of vaccines that were given routinely in the past. Tables 2.10 and 2.11 will help you make good decisions for your pet's vaccination needs and schedules.

Table 2.10 *Dog (Canine) Vaccinations Chart*

VACCINE	YOUNG PUPPIES	FINAL PUPPY VACCINES	FIRST VACCINE COMPLETED AT 16 WEEKS OR ONE YEAR OR OLDER	FIRST VACCINE AT ONE YEAR OR OLDER	VACCINE S GIVEN AT 16 WEEKS OR OLDER
PUPPY *Distemper* *Hepatitis* *(Adenovirus-2)* *& Parvovirus*	Start at 6 weeks of age repeat every 3-4 weeks until 12-14 weeks old	Final given at 16 or between 14 & 16 weeks	Repeat all vaccines in 1 year	One dose is considered to be protective	Revaccinate every 3 years
First vaccine at 16 Weeks *Distemper* *Hepatitis* *(Adenovirus-2)* *& Parvovirus*	1 year or 16 weeks of age	Repeat in 3-4 weeks is recommended but not considered essential	Repeat all vaccines in 1 year	One dose considered to be protective	Revaccinate every 3 years
Rabies	1 dose at 12 weeks or as required by state law		Repeat in 1 year	Repeat in 1 year	After 2nd immunization Revaccinate every 3 years
SPECIAL VACCINE FOR YOUNG DOGS ONLY					
Measles FOR YOUNG ONLY	Single Dose Between 6 & 12 weeks	Not Recommended	Not recommended	Not recommended	Not recommended

Leptospirosis, Canine parainfluenza, Bordetella, Borreliosis/Lyme disease, Canine coronavirus, & Giardia are considered to be noncore vaccines and given when required. Canine coronavirus and & Giardia are not recommended vaccines. Perhaps the most noncore vaccine used is Bordetella as it is often required when boarding a pet. **RABIES MAY BE REQUIRED BY LAW IN SOME STATES TO BE AN ANNUAL VACCINATION. THERE ARE ONE YEAR AND 3 YEAR VACCINES AVAILABLE**

Table 2.11 *Cat (Feline) Vaccinations Chart*

VACCINE	YOUNG OR NEW BORN KITTENS	VACCINES GIVEN AT 12 WEEKS OF AGE OR OLDER	FIRST KNOWN VACCINE GIVE AT 12 WEEKS OR 1 YEAR OF AGE	FIRST VACCINE GIVEN AT ONE YEAR OF AGE OR OLDER	ONE YEAR AFTER IMMUNIZATION SERIES OR AFTER 12 WEEK OR ONE YEAR VACCINE
Kitten FVRCP (Feline viral rhinotracheitis, calicivirus, panleukopenia)	Start immunizations series at 6 weeks of age repeat every 3-4 weeks. OR Repeat on weeks 8 & 11, Final at 12 weeks of age	Repeat in 1 year	Repeat in 3-4 weeks and again In 1 year	If immunization history is unknown immunize and repeat in 3-4 weeks and at 1 year then every 3 years. If previous vaccine history is known repeat every 3 years.	Repeat every 3 years. Make sure cat is getting 3 year vaccines and not 1 year vaccines
Rabies	Can be vaccinated ONLY if canarypox vaccine is used it is none adjuvanted	Repeat in 1 year	If first vaccination repeat in 1 year	If first vaccination repeat in 1 year and every 3 years there after	Repeat every 3 years. Make sure cat is getting 3 year vaccines and not 1 year vaccines

Feline leukemia, Feline immunodeficiency virus, Chlamydophila, Bordetella bronchiseptica & Giardia are noncore vaccines and not currently recommended for routine use, but may be used on selected case basis. Feline infectious peritonitis & Giardia are not recommended vaccines. Feline immunodeficiency virus vaccination is not recommended because it does not protect from all 5 FIV serotypes and confounds testing.

A word of thought on FIV: The FIV vaccine only protects for one of the five known serotypes of FIV. This makes FIV somewhat analogues to a human flu vaccine. The Center for Disease Control (CDC) selects the virus most apt to cause flu in our population and the flu vaccine is made with that virus serotype. The flu vaccine does not have all the serotypes of flu virus in the vaccine. If we are lucky and the virus that

CDC selects is correct we will not get the flu. If the CDC happens to be wrong and we get a different flu serotype we will get flu. So it is with FIV with only one serotype in the vaccine. If we are lucky and the serotype of FIV vaccinated for is the serotype FIV infection the cat gets then the cat will not get FIV. However, if the cat happens to contact one of the other four serotypes of FIV the cat.

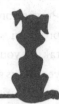

CHAPTER 3

WORMS, FLEAS, AND OTHER PARASITES

The difference between genius and stupidity is that genius has limits.
—Albert Einstein

Preventing parasitic diseases in people and pets has been a struggle throughout the history of mankind. Ancient Egyptian mummies have had blood flukes found in them. If one can prevent parasites, it makes everyone happy and saves frustration, fear, and money. There is no disease on the planet that is cheaper to treat than parasites. This chapter is about preventing and treating those nasty worms and other parasites that make our pets sick.

Our pets are a part of the family, and it is important to prevent parasite transmission from family members to pets and from pets to family members. In this chapter, there are many charts that enable one to have medication doses by weight of their pets at their fingertips. I asked many people if they want the chart next to the subject discussed or in an appendix. In an overwhelming response, they said they want it next to the conditions described. So it is. Therefore, some charts are repeated for this reason and you may see them more than once in this chapter. I hope pet parasite prevention and good health is as important to you as it is to me.

HEARTWORM PREVENTION

Heartworm prevention will save your pet from severe disease and save you big dollars since treatment for heartworms is very expensive. Prevention is consistent with my philosophy that a good wellness program will save you big bucks over a period of years. I recommend taking your pet to see the pet's doctor a minimum of two times per year. This allows for early diagnosis of disease conditions. If diagnosed early, things can normally be easier to treat. It has also resulted in preventing things from occurring or developing. Having said that, I know many folks will not take their pets to the pet's doctor. We will discuss how you can help prevent heartworms in your pet. The prevention is simple, but the treatment is very complex and very expensive. We will discuss a two-pronged attack to allow you to provide the best prevention you can with over-the-counter drugs.

Heartworms are transmitted by mosquitoes, and unfortunately there are several species of mosquitoes that do so. The larvae have to be in the mosquito at least three days before they can infect a pet. Unfortunately, this disease is worldwide. Alaska seems to have the fewest number of cases, and this is most likely due to the cold temperatures that occur and remain for at least a major portion of the year.

When a mosquito bites your dog, the mosquito injects heartworm larvae into your pet. The best heartworm-treatment plan is preventing mosquitoes from biting your pet. You can take steps to prevent mosquitoes from biting your pets by doing an inspection around your house to see if you have areas of standing water that can be used by mosquitoes for laying eggs. You might be surprised that many mosquitoes are coming from areas around your home due to small areas of stagnant water. Once you have found standing water, do what you can do to remove this type of mosquito-breeding areas near your home. Remember that it only takes a very small amount of water for mosquitoes to lay eggs and produce more mosquitoes. You might consider looking around your neighborhood for standing water too.

Another simple thing to do to help prevent heartworms in your dog is to use Advantix II. It is a Bayer Company product, and you can purchase this product online, at 1 (800) PetMeds, and in pet stores, such as Petco, PetSmart, and in many military PX and BX facilities. You need to use this product monthly. *You cannot treat once and think you have done your duty.* It just does not work that way.

Advantix II will treat fleas, mosquitoes, flies, ticks, and lice. It is a good product that is new to the market. It will also treat adult fleas, larvae, and flea eggs. You will be getting your money's worth with this product. However, you *must* use this product every month for the treatment to be effective or you will be wasting your time and money. Another benefit of this product is that it is waterproof. It will not wash off, and you can bathe your pet. All you have to do is put it on the back of the neck of your dog once per month—how simple is that?

Warning: Advantix II is not for use in cats. Cats do not have enzymes that can metabolize or degrade Advantix II, which results in poisoning (toxicity) in cats.

You can use 1 percent Ivermectin once per month by injecting the dose under the skin or by giving the dose by mouth. Either way is very effective, and it must be given once per month if you are to prevent heartworms. If you happen to miss a month, it will still be okay ,but you may no longer have a negative heartworm dog.

Table 3.1 gives you the necessary dosages for treating your pet. All you need to know is the weight of your pet to look up the dose to be given. The 1 percent Ivermectin can be purchased at feed stores. The 1 percent Ivermectin at feed stores is for large animals, such as pigs and cows, so make sure you purchase 1 percent Ivermectin for your use and use Table 3.1. *Do not overdose!* You do not want to introduce blindness, illness, or death. Look at the weight and get the correct dosage for your pet. The 1 percent Ivermectin at the chart dosages is safe for dogs and cats. You will be treating ear mites, lice, ticks, roundworms, hookworms, and scabies at the same time you are preventing heartworms.

If you give the Ivermectin by mouth, you can go online and look for "empty gelatin capsules." They are really cheap. You can put the Ivermectin in the gelatin capsules and help the medicine go down. This is not a necessary step, but it can be done to alleviate taste problems.

Some websites have different size capsules. If you click on the different sizes, it will let you know how much you can put into the capsule. You can also make a small pocket in some ground beef or another soft food; put the Ivermectin in it and let the pet woof it down. Cats do not normally woof them down.

TREATMENT

Treatment can be accomplished by using a monthly dose for an indefinite period of time. This is considered to be a slow method of treatment, which has fallen from favor, but it is an effective treatment over time. See Table 3.1; look up your pet's weight and obtain the dose for your pet's weight. The 1 percent Ivermection can be purchased at feed stores or tractor stores.

PREVENTION

This entire presentation has been about prevention—all of which you can do. If you happen to forget a month, you are still okay, but you must not miss the next treatment. The best diagnostic tools for determining if a pet is heartworm positive is via an antigen test. The most sensitive test to date is the so-called snap test [ELISA], but any antigen test that will test for heartworms is good. However, it only tests for female worms. Currently there is no test that will detect an all-male worm infection. If your pet ever tests positive for heartworms, it is sure to have the disease since the tests are very sensitive and accurate. Annual screening is highly recommended; your pet's doctor can do this for you or you can have it done at an immunization clinic, such as Luv My Pet. Use of such clinics might be cheaper.

Table 3.1 1 Percent Ivermectin Dose-by-Weight Chart

(weight divided by 80 = dose in cc)

Weight Pounds	Dose cc	Weight Pounds	Dose cc	Weight Pounds	Dose cc	Weight Pounds	Dose cc	Weight Pounds	Dose cc
1	0.01	21	0.26	41	0.51	61	0.76	81	1.01
2	0.02	22	0.27	42	0.52	62	0.77	82	1.02
3	0.03	23	0.28	43	0.53	63	0.78	83	1.03
4	0.05	24	0.30	44	0.55	64	0.80	84	1.05
5	0.06	25	0.31	45	0.56	65	0.81	85	1.06
6	0.07	26	0.32	46	0.57	66	0.82	86	1.07
7	0.08	27	0.33	47	0.58	67	0.83	87	1.08
8	0.10	28	0.35	48	0.60	68	0.85	88	1.10
9	0.11	29	0.36	49	0.61	69	0.86	89	1.11
10	0.12	30	0.37	50	0.62	70	0.87	90	1.12
11	0.13	31	0.38	51	0.63	71	0.88	91	1.13
12	0.15	32	0.40	52	0.65	72	0.90	92	1.15
13	0.16	33	0.41	53	0.66	73	0.91	93	1.16
14	0.17	34	0.42	54	0.67	74	0.92	94	1.17
15	0.18	35	0.43	55	0.68	75	0.93	95	1.18
16	0.20	36	0.45	56	0.70	76	0.95	96	1.20
17	0.21	37	0.46	57	0.71	77	0.96	97	1.21
18	0.22	38	0.47	58	0.72	78	0.97	98	1.22
19	0.23	39	0.49	59	0.73	79	0.98	99	1.23
20	0.25	40	0.50	60	0.75	80	1.00	100	1.25

PARASITE TIME FROM EXPOSURE TO INFECTION

Clients ask, "When my pet is exposed to XYZ parasite, how long until there is an infection that can be seen in my pet?"

The time frame from exposure to signs of infection is most commonly called the "prepatent period." The definition of prepatent period in parasitology is "the period equivalent to the incubation period of microbial infections." Of course, the pet has the parasite before it can be seen or diagnosed because many of the parasites have a migration phase in the pet's body before it shows up in the intestines. The time during which the disease process has begun but is not yet clinically manifested is called the "prodromal period." Table 3.2 shows the parasites' common names, scientific names, and time until the disease can be diagnosed and/or seen:

Table 3.2 *Parasite Time from Exposure to Infection*

Infective Worms	Animals Infected	Time from Infection until Clinical Signs	Over-the-Counter Treatment Purchase at Feed Stores
Roundworms [Ascrids]			
Toxocara canis +	Dogs	4–5 weeks	Panacur
Toxocara cati ++	Cats	6–8 weeks	Panacur
Toxascaris leonine	Dogs and cats	Approx. 10 weeks	Panacur
Hookworms			
Ancylostoma canium ingestion	Dogs	2 weeks	Panacur
Transcutaneous [through the skin]	Dogs	4 weeks	Panacur
Uncinara stenocephala Ingestion	Dogs and cats	2–2.5 weeks	Panacur
Transcutaneous [through the skin]	Dogs and cats	4 weeks	Panacur
Ancylostoma tubaeforme	Cats		
Ingestion	Cats	2.5–3 weeks	Panacur
Transcutaneous [through the skin]	Cats	4 weeks	Panacur
Whipworms			
Trichuris vulpis	Dogs	12–13 weeks	Panacur

Tapeworms			
Taenia pisiformis	Dogs	6–8 weeks	Panacur
Taenia taeniaeformis	Cats	5–11 weeks	Panacur
Echinococcus granulosus	Dogs	6–9 weeks	Panacur
Echinococcus multilocularis	Dogs and cats	4–5 weeks	Panacur
Dipylidium caninum	Dogs and cats	2–3 weeks	Panacur

+ = pre- and postnatal for T. Canis 2–3 weeks. ++ = postnatal for T. Cati 6 weeks

FLEA ALLERGY DERMATITIS

Flea allergy is caused by an owner not treating the pet for fleas. As the flea bites, it injects half of a protein into the body. This half joins with half a protein in the body, and this combination sets the stage for the allergy. The good news is that it can be prevented by simply treating the pet with a flea product. You need to make sure the product you purchase is a quality product that will work. Many cheap products are good for spending money—but are not great for treating fleas. Many new products for treating fleas are great and easy to use. All you have to do is put the flea meds on the skin of the dog—not the hair. I suggest Advantage II for cats and young dogs, and Advantix II for dogs only, which also treats for mosquitoes and ticks.

Once the pet gets a flea allergy, it only takes one flea bite—and the dog starts to scratch. The bad news is that once the dog has the allergy, it takes a rather lengthy time to treat and get all the hair that has been lost to grow back in.

The bad news continues once the allergy is established. It is an opportunity for skin infections caused by bacteria and fungi. Unfortunately, skin infections are common secondary responses to flea allergies, and most skin damage is due to the pet biting and chewing at the skin caused by a flea bites.

If you have not been treating for fleas—but have now started to treat your pet—remember to be persistent and consistent with the flea treatment or you will never get the pet well. By now, you know it is so much cheaper to prevent disease than to treat disease. Get that medicine for fleas before it is too late.

A lady came in to have her dog spayed, and she commented that she was using Benadryl to keep the dog from scratching, but it was not effective. While doing the surgery, it was noted that the dog had a very heavy infestation of fleas. It was no wonder the dog was scratching. The poor creature was loaded with fleas. You have to treat the cause of the disease—not the signs of any disease—or you will never be successful with your treatments.

TREATMENT

The treatment of flea allergy dermatitis is to treat for fleas constantly and persistently until all the hair grows back in—and then treat forever to prevent hair loss from reoccurring. You can obtain Advantage II for cats and Advantix II for dogs. These products need to be used monthly; if there is a really bad infestation of fleas, it may be necessary to treat every two weeks for a period of time.

These products can be purchased at PetSmart 1 (800) PetMeds, Petco, and most military PX and BX stores. Your pet's doctor will have flea medications also. If you purchase large-dog products, you can give the dosage for the flea treatment in this chapter under the article "A Low-Cost Treatment for Fleas." It will save you some money. If the pet has mutilated itself due to biting and scratching, the wounds need to be treated as well.

PREVENTION

Many areas in the United States and Canada have problems with fleas, and the only thing we have available to prevent fleas is the constant treatment of pets. Consistent and persistent treatment for fleas will ensure that the pests are defeated before they get started on your pet.

Those of you who live in higher elevations do not have flea problems due to the lower temperatures. You're the lucky ones when it comes to this disease. You can purchase flea prevention and treatments online, in pet stores, at some military PX and BX stores, and at Walmart. We use Advantage II on small dogs and cats and Advantix II on larger dogs because the products work and are effective against flea, flea eggs, and flea larvae. If you have fleas or think you have fleas in your house, one of the best ways to remove them is to use a flea trap. You can obtain a flea trap online at www. myfleatrap.com. The trap is chemical-free and simple to use. Simple instructions come with the trap.

I loaned my flea trap to one of the ladies who works at our facility, and it was so effective that she purchased two of her own traps. If you use the trap and do not catch any fleas, you do not have fleas in the house. If there are fleas in the house, the trap will catch them. It is very effective.

FLEAS

Fleas are one of the most common causes of scratching and biting of the body for dogs and cats. In fact,
many people treat the scratching and are concerned
about other skin conditions, and it is more commonly due
to fleas.

Treat for fleas first and get good flea control before putting money into skin conditions. It is an unhappy experience to learn late in the game when you find out that the pet has had fleas all along—and the pet has not been properly treated for fleas. Recently we have had dogs with so many fleas that the dogs were very anemic due to the loss of blood caused by the fleas.

Fleas are most prevalent during periods of rain and hot weather. Higher elevations are not plagued with fleas due to the lower temperatures. One of the most common sources of fleas is wildlife bringing fleas into yards at night. Before the sun comes up, it is not uncommon to see raccoons or possums roaming from house to house. Fleas tend to be found in shaded areas and *not* in areas that get lots of sunshine. Heavy infestations of fleas are found under bushes, decks, and large shade trees. These areas need to be treated for fleas. If you treat or are having your yard treated, it is considered a waste of time and money to spray where the yard gets lots of sunshine.

Although there are many different species of fleas, the most common ones on cats is *Ctenocephalides felis* and for dogs *Ctenocephalides canis*. They cause little red dots of irritation on the abdomen of cats and dogs and are a very common sign of fleas. Fleas tend to be more prevalent in the area just in front of where the tail hooks onto the body (the tail head).

An easy way to diagnose fleas is to put a 3x5 card behind and next to the tail head. Scratch the dander and debris onto the card; little black specks will often be seen on the card. Wet your hand and let a few drops of water drop onto the card; you will often see red streaks from the little black dots. The little black dots are flea feces, which is dried blood. The drops of water you let drip from your hand dissolve the black specks of dry blood, and you will see streaks of red blood. When you see the red streaks, you have your diagnosis of fleas. This is a fast, effective way to diagnose fleas. A good treatment is Advantix II (dogs) or Advantage II (dogs and cats) available online, at pet stores, and at many military PX or BX facilities.

TREATMENT

I recommend Advantage II for cats and Advantix II for dogs. Both products are available at pet stores, military BX and PX facilities, and Walmart. Advantage II is designed for dog and cats, but you can purchase the product for a dog or a cat. Advantix II is for dogs only. We have used these products on thousands of dogs and cats without any problems. We use them as the manufacturer recommends. Areas where flea meds have been placed on a pet will become hairless. I have no good reason for why this happens, but the good news is that it is a rare occurrence. The bad news is that it is disturbing to owners when it happens.

PREVENTION

Prevention of fleas is simple—just treat your pet once a month forever. I have learned that many people will treat their pets every three or six months. This type of treatment is asking for flea allergy dermatitis to develop. Treating every month is very important if you want to prevent flea infestations in your pets.

HAIR LOSS DUE TO DEMODEX MITES

Hair loss is a common issue with pets, and many things can be the cause. Here we will discuss hair loss caused by demodex mites. Demodex mites are small bugs that live in hair follicles or root areas of hairs. These mites cause an area of hair to be lost and can cause even more skin issues and skin infections.

Skin infections are commonly associated with demodex mite infestations that are allowed to become chronic infections. Hair loss due to demodex can be localized or generalized; neither is wanted by pet owners. The mites are said to be present on normal healthy pets, but their excellent immune systems keep them from having any hair loss due to the mites.

Demodex is the cause of the common skin condition known as "Red Mange." Unfortunately, the red skin condition is an advanced state of the disease, and it is not good to allow this to happen to your pet. The localized type of hair loss can be a single small area of hair loss or multiple areas of hair loss. It is more common in younger dogs, but small demodex hair loss can be found in dogs of any age.

Localized lesions are normally treated with a topical product containing benzoyl peroxide. If this does not work, Ivermectin is normally the treatment of choice. When generalized hair loss is more extensive or infected, the skin may have an odor associated with the hair loss. Once smelled, you will not forget it. You will be able to easily identify the demodex odor in the future since it has a very pungent, distinct smell. If you smell this odor, you are definitely doing something wrong. The diagnosis is made by scraping the skin, placing it in mineral oil on a microscope slide, and looking at it with a microscope. You may need your pet's doctor to make the diagnosis for you.

The cigar-shaped mites have eight legs (see image), and they are not anything that one wants on their pet.

TREATMENT

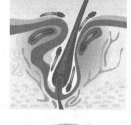

Demodex can be a very difficult disease to treat, but if you are persistent with the treatment, the dog will improve—and the odor and hair will return to normal. Tables 3.3, 3.4, and 3.5 show the dosage for day one, day two, and all other treatments. All you need to know is your pet's weight; you can use Tables 3.3, 3.4, and 3.5 to find the dose you need.

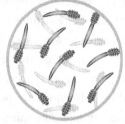

Caution: Do not overdose! It can cause blindness and central nervous system issues if you give too much. Use Tables 3.3, 3.4, and 3.5. You can purchase 1 percent Ivermectin at feed stores. The product is labeled for cattle and pigs, but it is effective for all species and depends on proper dosing to prevent any overdose issues. When you purchase the Ivermectin, make sure it is a 1 percent solution or the chart below will not be correct. Tables 3.3, 3.4, and 3.5 are good for all animals—not just dogs and cats—provided the animal is not allergic to Ivermectin.

RABBITS

Ivermectin does a nice job on rabbit ear mites as well. Use the dose by weight of the rabbit that is found in Table 3.1 and give the correct weight dose to the rabbit: one dose initially, then another dose two weeks later. If necessary a third dose can be added in two weeks. Do not remove the accumulated material on the ears generated by the ear mite, as it will fall away by itself due to the treatment.

PREVENTION

Unfortunately, we do not yet know how to prevent this disease from occurring. It normally occurs spontaneously and often is not noticed until there is enough hair loss to cause concern.

Table 3.3 *Day 1 Demodex Dose-by-Weight Chart*

1 Percent Ivermectin Dosing Chart
(weight divided by 100 = dose in cc)

Weight Pounds	Dose cc	Weight Pounds	Dose cc	Weight Pounds	Dose cc	Weight Pounds	Dose cc	Weight Pounds	Dose cc
1	0.01	21	0.21	41	0.41	61	0.61	81	0.81
2	0.02	22	0.22	42	0.42	62	0.62	82	0.82
3	0.03	23	0.23	43	0.43	63	0.63	83	0.83
4	0.04	24	0.24	44	0.44	64	0.64	84	0.84
5	0.05	25	0.25	45	0.45	65	0.65	85	0.85
6	0.06	26	0.26	46	0.46	66	0.66	86	0.86
7	0.07	27	0.27	47	0.47	67	0.67	87	0.87
8	0.08	28	0.28	48	0.48	68	0.68	88	0.88
9	0.09	29	0.29	49	0.49	69	0.69	89	0.89
10	0.10	30	0.30	50	0.50	70	0.70	90	0.90
11	0.11	31	0.31	51	0.51	71	0.71	91	0.91
12	0.12	32	0.32	52	0.52	72	0.72	92	0.92
13	0.13	33	0.33	53	0.53	73	0.73	93	0.93
14	0.14	34	0.34	54	0.54	74	0.74	94	0.94
15	0.15	35	0.35	55	0.55	75	0.75	95	0.95
16	0.16	36	0.36	56	0.56	76	0.76	96	0.96
17	0.17	37	0.37	57	0.57	77	0.77	97	0.97
18	0.18	38	0.38	58	0.58	78	0.78	98	0.98
19	0.19	39	0.39	59	0.59	79	0.79	99	0.99
20	0.20	40	0.40	60	0.60	80	0.80	100	1.00

Table 3.4 *Day 2 Demodex Dose-by-Weight Chart*

1 Percent Ivermectin Dosing Chart
(2 times per day, 1 dose = dose in cc)

Weight Pounds	Dose cc	Weight Pounds	Dose cc	Weight Pounds	Dose cc	Weight Pounds	Dose cc	Weight Pounds	Dose cc
1	0.02	21	0.42	41	0.82	61	1.22	81	1.62
2	0.04	22	0.44	42	0.84	62	1.24	82	1.64
3	0.06	23	0.46	43	0.86	63	1.26	83	1.66
4	0.08	24	0.48	44	0.88	64	1.28	84	1.68
5	0.10	25	0.50	45	0.90	65	1.30	85	1.70
6	0.12	26	0.52	46	0.92	66	1.32	86	1.72
7	0.14	27	0.54	47	0.94	67	1.34	87	1.74
8	0.16	28	0.56	48	0.96	68	1.36	88	1.76
9	0.18	29	0.58	49	0.98	69	1.38	89	1.78
10	0.20	30	0.60	50	1.00	70	1.40	90	1.80
11	0.22	31	0.62	51	1.02	71	1.42	91	1.82
12	0.24	32	0.64	52	1.04	72	1.44	92	1.84
13	0.26	33	0.66	53	1.06	73	1.46	93	1.86
14	0.28	34	0.68	54	1.08	74	1.48	94	1.88
15	0.30	35	0.70	55	1.10	75	1.50	95	1.90
16	0.32	36	0.72	56	1.12	76	1.52	96	1.92
17	0.34	37	0.74	57	1.14	77	1.54	97	1.94
18	0.36	38	0.76	58	1.16	78	1.56	98	1.96
19	0.38	39	0.78	59	1.18	79	1.58	99	1.98
20	0.40	40	0.80	60	1.20	80	1.60	100	2.00

Table 3.5 *Days 3-14 (Maybe More) Demodex Dose-by-Weight Chart*

1 Percent Ivermectin Dosing Chart
(day-1 dose times 3 = dose in cc)

Weight Pounds	Dose cc	Weight Pounds	Dose cc	Weight Pounds	Dose cc	Weight Pounds	Dose cc	Weight Pounds	Dose cc
1	0.03	21	0.63	41	1.23	61	1.83	81	2.43
2	0.06	22	0.66	42	1.26	62	1.86	82	2.46
3	0.09	23	0.69	43	1.29	63	1.89	83	2.49
4	0.12	24	0.72	44	1.32	64	1.92	84	2.52
5	0.15	25	0.75	45	1.35	65	1.95	85	2.55
6	0.18	26	0.78	46	1.38	66	1.98	86	2.58
7	0.21	27	0.81	47	1.41	67	2.01	87	2.61
8	0.24	28	0.84	48	1.44	68	2.04	88	2.64
9	0.27	29	0.87	49	1.47	69	2.07	89	2.67
10	0.30	30	0.90	50	1.50	70	2.10	90	2.70
11	0.33	31	0.93	51	1.53	71	2.13	91	2.73
12	0.36	32	0.96	52	1.56	72	2.16	92	2.76
13	0.39	33	0.99	53	1.59	73	2.19	93	2.79
14	0.42	34	1.02	54	1.62	74	2.22	94	2.82
15	0.45	35	1.05	55	1.65	75	2.25	95	2.85
16	0.48	36	1.08	56	1.68	76	2.28	96	2.88
17	0.51	37	1.11	57	1.71	77	2.31	97	2.91
18	0.54	38	1.14	58	1.74	78	2.34	98	2.94
19	0.57	39	1.17	59	1.77	79	2.37	99	2.97
20	0.60	40	1.20	60	1.80	80	2.40	100	3.00

A LOW-COST TREATMENT FOR FLEAS

Fleas are a common skin problem for pets in most areas of the United States and Canada. However, if you live in a higher elevation, fleas cannot survive—and you're the lucky ones when it comes to fleas. Areas of the country that get lots of rain and lots of hot weather are ideal for flea populations. These areas have the highest concentration of fleas, and they tend to be a year-round problem for pets.

We recently had a lady bring in her dog for surgery. She was giving Benadryl to help keep the poor dog from scratching. We found the dog was covered in fleas. Therefore, the Benadryl was a waste of money and time. This is a very important point about treating your pet. One *must* treat the condition—and not the signs of the condition—if one expects to be successful with any treatment for any condition. Another simple example of treating signs and not the condition would be giving pain pills to a pet for a broken leg and expecting the pet to get well. The pain pills will not fix the leg.

There are new medications on the market for fleas, and we like to use Advantage II for dogs and cats and Advantix II for dogs only. Both of these products can be purchased at pet stores, such as Petco, PetSmart, and Walmart, and at military PX and BX stores. If you purchase these products, you need to buy the product according to the weight of your pet.

I have been told by clients that they buy the large Advantage II product. I have been asked what to do if they purchase the large dose of Advantage II. At our facility, we purchase the large Advantage II and pour it into a small plastic bottle—and then we give a dose for fleas according to the dosage chart below (Table 3.6). We have treated thousands of animals using the dosages in Table 3.6. Some animals are so infested with fleas that they need a second dose. We wait a day or two and repeat. Remember to apply the medication to the back of the neck, making sure it is put on the skin and not just on the hair.

Table 3.6 *Low-Cost Flea Treatment Dosages*

Dogs
Advantage II
Less than 4 weeks of age = 0.1 cc
Between 4–7 weeks of age = 0.2 cc
Dogs greater than 7 weeks of age
0–10 pounds = 0.4 cc
11–20 pounds = 1.0 cc
21–50 pounds = 2.5 cc
51–100—pounds = 4.0 cc

Cats
Canine Advantage II
Less than 4 weeks of age = 0.1 cc
Between 4–7 weeks of age = 0.2 cc
Cats greater than four weeks of age
0–9 pounds = 0.4 cc
9+ pounds = 0.8 cc

Activyl is a new flea medication that is available from veterinarians. If you purchase this product in the largest dose, you can dose your pets according to the following charts:

Dogs
Activyl
4–14 pounds = 0.51 cc
14–22 pounds = 0.77 cc
22–44 pounds = 1.54 cc
44–88 pounds = 3.08 cc
88–132 pounds = 4.62 cc

Cats
Activyl
2–9 pounds = 0.51 cc
9+ pounds = 1.03 cc

CAT TOXOPLASMOSIS INFECTIONS AND YOU

Unfortunately, toxoplasmosis is ubiquitous. It seems to be everywhere, and this organism infects all mammals, including people. Toxoplasmosis seems to complete its entire life cycle in cats only. Cats spread the disease via the feces they deposit. The organism is very resistant to the environment and chemicals and survives for very long periods of time.

Dogs can pass the organism in their feces if they accidentally or intentionally eat cat feces. Basically, the signs of toxoplasmosis are similar to many other diseases. Therefore, diagnosis of the condition is best left to the pet's doctor. None of the signs caused by the infection of toxoplasmosis documents the disease; diagnosis will require special testing.

The disease organism is known as *Toxoplasma gondii* and can only be identified in feces by a fecal flotation exam, in tissues prepared for observation under a microscope, or by serology testing. Cats tend not to be feces eaters [coprophagic] and obtain the disease by eating small rodents and other small animals.

Toxoplasmosis can infect dogs. Dogs and all other infected mammals are considered intermediate hosts. An intermediate host is a mammal with the organism in its body from some source, and it will infect any other mammal that eats it or any parts of the mammal. This is another good reason for chefs to cook meats well before eating them.

According to the CDC, toxoplasmosis is the leading cause of death in people from foodborne illness in the United States. The CDC also puts the number of toxoplasmosis-infected men, women, and children in the United States at 60 million (Centers for Disease Control and Prevention, Atlanta, GA). Infection can also occur if a mammal happens to obtain oral contamination from cat feces infected with toxoplasmosis. Toxoplasmosis can spread to neonatal animals, including people, during pregnancy and cause stillborn young. Approximately 30–40 percent of cats and 20 percent of dogs in the United States tend to test positive or have seropositive tests—and therefore are presumed to be infected with toxoplasmosis.

TREATMENT

There are no over-the-counter drugs that can be obtained that will treat this disease.

PREVENTION

This can be tricky since it is difficult or impossible to control outdoor cats and keep them from eating small animals in the outdoors. Indoor cats that are never let out are considered quarantined for all intents and purposes. Indoor cats are least likely to become infected with toxoplasmosis. People cleaning cat litter should be aware of the need for caution when disposing of cat litter—and it may be wise to use disposable gloves. It is often advised that pregnant women should not clean cat litter at all until after delivery. There are medical reports indicating that large populations of people have obtained brain infections of toxoplasmosis, which may be a cause of some mental disorders.

THE NEED FOR ROUTINE FECAL EXAMS

Routine fecal exams are an essential part of keeping your pet healthy. I recommend that a pet see the doctor on a wellness program at least two times per year; if you do this, your pet will routinely have fecal exams. If you do not take your pet to see the doctor twice per year, you should take a fecal sample in to have it examined for internal parasites twice per year—or at least once per year.

Dogs and cats can become infected with internal parasites, which can cause anemia and death. Parasites are easy to treat, and you can prevent unnecessary health conditions and potential death. Unfortunately, I see way too many dogs and cats that have internal parasites. Some dogs have weight loss and bloody, loose stools, and/or diarrhea from anemia. This can be prevented by having routine internal parasite exams and treating for internal parasites on a routine basis. Some parasites in dogs and cats can cause health conditions for the pet owners. Internal parasites are easy to treat; there is no excuse for unhealthy pets due to parasites.

There are many compounds that can be used for treating internal parasites. Some flea medications, such as Revolution, will kill internal parasites and prevent heartworms in dogs and cats. Revolution requires a prescription and does a good job. However, you can purchase a bottle of Panacur with a concentration of 100 mg per cc at a feed store and give 25 mg per pound of body weight. See Table 3.7 for dose by weight for dogs and cats.

When you find the dose on Table 3.7 for your pet, use that dose for three consecutive days. Follow-up treatment needs to be done for an additional three days two weeks later. Panacur is a large-animal product and comes in a rather large plastic bottle that will last for a long time. Make sure you shake it well before taking any medication from the bottle. Panacur is available in smaller amounts at 1 (800) PetMeds, pet stores, PetSmart, and Petco.

TREATMENT

Panacur is an easy product to use for internal parasites, and it will remove all internal parasites from the intestines. Use Table 3.7 to find the correct dosage. Give this dose for three days and repeat the dosage in two weeks for three days to get the worms that were in the migration phase of infestation.

Panacur is available at feed stores. If you purchase Panacur at the feed store, be sure to purchase 100 mg/cc Panacur to enable you to use the chart below. Or you can purchase Panacur at pet stores such as PetSmart, Petco, and at 1 (800) PetMeds. If you purchase at these stores, follow the directions on the containers.

PREVENTION

Parasites are easy for pets to acquire. They can be born with roundworms or get worms from the milk of the mother. Any pet that is allowed outside can become infected. Prevention of diseases from parasites can be accomplished by routine fecal checks at your veterinarian or anywhere there is a centrifuge and a microscope. Panacur will treat roundworms, hookworms, tapeworms, giardia, liver flukes, and other parasites. Due to the numerous worms treated with Panacur, it becomes a medicine of choice. Your goal is to always have negative fecal exams. This is accomplished by having fecal tests run on a routine basis and proper treatment when necessary.

Table 3.7 *Panacur (Fenbendazole) Dose-by-Weight Chart*

100 mg/cc Panacur [Fenbendazole] Dosing Chart
Repeat the dose for three days and then repeat
the three-day treatment in two weeks.
(weight times 25 divided by 100 = dose in cc)

Weight Pounds	Dose cc	Weight Pounds	Dose cc	Weight Pounds	Dose cc	Weight Pounds	Dose cc	Weight Pounds	Dose cc
1	0.25	21	5.25	41	10.25	61	15.25	81	20.25
2	0.50	22	5.50	42	10.50	62	15.50	82	20.50
3	0.75	23	5.75	43	10.75	63	15.75	83	20.75
4	1.0	24	6.0	44	11.00	64	16.0	84	21.0
5	1.25	25	6.25	45	11.25	65	16.25	85	21.25
6	1.50	26	6.50	46	11.50	66	16.50	86	21.50
7	1.75	27	6.75	47	11.75	67	16.75	87	21.75
8	2.0	28	7.0	48	12.0	68	17.0	88	22.0
9	2.25	29	7.25	49	12.25	69	17.25	89	22.25
10	2.50	30	7.50	50	12.50	70	17.50	90	22.50
11	2.75	31	7.75	51	12.75	71	17.75	91	22.75
12	3.00	32	8.0	52	13.0	72	18.0	92	23.0
13	3.25	33	8.25	53	13.25	73	18.25	93	23.25
14	3.50	34	8.50	54	13.50	74	18.50	94	23.50
15	3.75	35	8.75	55	13.75	75	18.75	95	23.75
16	4.00	36	9.0	56	14.0	76	19.0	96	24.0
17	4.25	37	9.25	57	14.25	77	19.25	97	24.25
18	4.50	38	9.50	58	14.50	78	19.50	98	24.50
19	4.75	39	9.75	59	14.75	79	19.75	99	24.75
20	5.00	40	10.0	60	15.0	80	20.0	100	25.0

MY PET KEEPS SCRATCHING

"My pet keeps scratching" is the most common complaint I hear from pet owners who are treating their pets for fleas. There are several causes that might be underlying issues with this syndrome. Let's focus on some of the things that *might* be the cause of this problem.

The leading reason is an infrequent treatment schedule for fleas. The manufacturers of flea medications call for monthly treatments. However, when I ask the question of those who have difficulty with continual flea problems, they cannot remember when they last treated for fleas. Most often, the pet has been treated once in a year or every six months—or maybe if the pet is lucky every three months. Many are too embarrassed to answer the question. No medical treatments on the planet will treat any animal for fleas beyond a month. In heavy flea areas, it is necessary to treat every two weeks to keep control of fleas.

Another reason your pet may still be scratching is that a flea-infested pet who resides inside the house causes the home to become plagued with fleas. It is a never-ending cycle. We were told in veterinary college that for every flea on the pet, there are probably a hundred in the house. I am not sure about the actual numbers, but it is true about fleas infesting the house.

Fleas lay their eggs on pets. The eggs fall off onto the carpets, couches, chairs, beds, and other furniture and develop into larvae and then into fleas. We have a client who has fleas on her pets and in her house. She said the treatment is doing no good. I offered her one of my flea traps. She caught so many fleas that she bought two more flea traps of her own. She swears by the flea traps and is starting to get control of the house and her pets. The flea trap has worked extremely well in combating her flea problem. The trap can be purchased online at www.myfleatrap.com. The trap is easy to use and works extremely well. This trap can also be purchased at Amazon.com.

There are several brands of flea traps, and my limited experience is with the flea trap that is available from Westham Innovations Company. Their telephone number is 1-888-722-3069. As for the other home flea trap companies you may see on Amazon.com, I have no idea about their effectiveness since I have not used them. If you catch no fleas, then you have no fleas in your house. If you do catch fleas, be aware that you will have several fleas in your trap and in your house.

If you have not treated at all or you have treated so infrequently, your pet might develop flea allergy dermatitis. Flea allergies are discussed in this book. Some pet owners treat for signs of flea infestation instead of the disease. For example, a pet owner may be administering Benadryl for scratching and the poor animal is loaded with fleas. Benadryl will not, has not, and will never treat fleas.

Fleas like to hang out in shaded areas of trees, bushes, or under decks. The pet will become infested with fleas all over again. Pets can have so many fleas that they acquire anemia or lack of blood in their body. Do not let this happen to your pets—and treat them correctly for fleas.

TREATMENT

My favorite treatment for fleas is Revolution. Revolution requires a prescription and can be purchased at 1 (800) PetMeds or from your veterinarian. New products are on the market. Our shelter uses Advantage II and Advantix II. Advantage II can be purchased for cats and dogs. Advantix II is designed for dogs only. Do not use Advantix II on cats.

You can purchase Advantage II for cats and dogs or Advantix II for dogs only at Petco, PetSmart, online, at many military PX and BX stores, and at feed stores. Remember to treat your pet at least once per month.

PREVENTION

Treat for fleas every month at a minimum.

COCCIDIA

Coccidia are intestinal parasites that invade cells of the lining of the intestines and multiply in the cells. The coccidia multiply until they cause the cells to burst open and spew new coccidia into the lumen or the middle of the intestines. These new coccidia invade more intestinal lining cells and repeat the process. The cells bursting open due to the coccidia reproducing in cells lining the small intestines cause the cells to burst, which creates bleeding within the intestinal tract. These events set the stage for diarrhea to develop. Coccidiosis leads to dehydration, loss of electrolytes, weight loss, acute anemia, weakness, and ultimately can lead to death. This disease is common in young kittens and puppies.

The sooner the diagnosis of the cause of the diarrhea can be made, the sooner it can be treated to prevent any further damage to the intestines. The best way to determine the cause is to obtain a fecal sample and have it checked for parasites. Coccidia and hookworms will cause bloody diarrhea and add to the need for proper diagnosis and proper and quick treatment. It is important that diarrhea is kept in its perspective since there are many conditions that will produce diarrhea quickly and severely.

TREATMENT

Without the equipment to run a fecal float and a microscope to examine the fecal float, it is impossible to know if one is actually treating coccidia. Therefore, this disease is best left to the pet's doctor for diagnosis and treatment. Treatment can be done blind without harm, but the drug costs money—and if it is not needed, you have wasted your money.

For individuals who insist on treating their pets, see Tables 3.8. and 3.9. Sulmet comes in a rather large container, and you will have enough Sulfadimethoxine to treat a battalion of pets for years. Sulmet is designed to be used in water for chicken coccidia. You can get medication from the pet's doctor or get a prescription from your veterinarian and purchase Albon online. Albon comes in liquid and tablet form. If you purchase Albon (Sulfadimethoxine), follow the directions on the container.

PREVENTION

Feed and water utensils should be cleaned and not allowed to become contaminated with fecal matter. This is a fecal oral infestation disease and avoiding contact with animals that have coccidia is the best thing you can do.

Table 3.8 *Dog and Cat Day 1 Sulmet (Sulfadimethoxine) Dose-by-Weight Chart*

12.5 Percent Sulmet (Sulfadimethoxine 125 mg/cc)
(weight divided by 5 = dose in cc)

Administer by mouth only. *If desired, dilute with water and double the volume.*

Weight Pounds	Dose cc	Weight Pounds	Dose cc	Weight Pounds	Dose cc	Weight Pounds	Dose cc	Weight Pounds	Dose cc
1	0.2	21	4.2	41	8.2	61	12.2	81	16.2
2	0.4	22	4.4	42	8.4	62	12.4	82	16.4
3	0.6	23	4.6	43	8.6	63	12.6	83	16.6
4	0.8	24	4.8	44	8.8	64	12.8	84	16.8
5	1.0	25	5.0	45	9.0	65	13.0	85	17.0
6	1.2	26	5.2	46	9.2	66	13.2	86	17.2
7	1.4	27	5.4	47	9.4	67	13.4	87	17.4
8	1.6	28	5.6	48	9.6	68	13.6	88	17.6
9	1.8	29	5.8	49	9.8	69	13.8	89	17.8
10	2.0	30	6.0	50	10	70	14.0	90	18.0
11	2.2	31	6.2	51	10.2	71	14.2	91	18.2
12	2.4	32	6.4	52	10.4	72	14.4	92	18.4
13	2.6	33	6.6	53	10.6	73	14.6	93	18.6
14	2.8	34	6.8	54	10.8	74	14.8	94	18.8
15	3.0	35	7.0	55	11.0	75	15.0	95	19.0
16	3.2	36	7.2	56	11.2	76	15.2	96	19.2
17	3.4	37	7.4	57	11.4	77	15.4	97	19.4
18	3.6	38	7.6	58	11.6	78	15.6	98	19.6
19	3.8	39	7.8	59	11.8	79	15.8	99	19.8
20	4.0	40	8.0	60	12.0	80	16.0	100	2.0

Table 3.9 Dog and Cat Days 2-5 Sulmet (Sulfadimethoxine) Dose-by-Weight Chart

12.5 Percent Sulmet (Sulfadimethoxine 125 mg/cc)
(divide day-1 dose by 2 = dose in cc)
Give by mouth only.
If desired, dilute with water and double the volume.

Weight Pounds	Dose cc	Weight Pounds	Dose cc	Weight Pounds	Dose cc	Weight Pounds	Dose cc	Weight Pounds	Dose cc
1	0.1	21	2.1	41	4.1	61	6.1	81	8.1
2	0.2	22	2.2	42	4.2	62	6.2	82	8.2
3	0.3	23	2.3	43	4.3	63	6.3	83	8.3
4	0.4	24	2.4	44	4.4	64	6.4	84	8.4
5	0.5	25	2.5	45	4.5	65	6.5	85	8.5
6	0.6	26	2.6	46	4.6	66	6.6	86	8.6
7	0.7	27	2.7	47	4.7	67	6.7	87	8.7
8	0.8	28	2.8	48	4.8	68	6.8	88	8.8
9	0.9	29	2.9	49	4.9	69	6.9	89	8.9
10	1.0	30	3.0	50	5.0	70	7.0	90	9.0
11	1.1	31	3.1	51	5.1	71	7.1	91	9.1
12	1.2	32	3.2	52	5.2	72	7.2	92	9.2
13	1.3	33	3.3	53	5.3	73	7.3	93	9.3
14	1.4	34	3.4	54	5.4	74	7.4	94	9.4
15	1.5	35	3.5	55	5.5	75	7.5	95	9.5
16	1.6	36	3.6	56	5.6	76	7.6	96	9.6
17	1.7	37	3.7	57	5.7	77	7.7	97	9.7
18	1.8	38	3.8	58	5.8	78	7.8	98	9.8
19	1.9	39	3.9	59	5.9	79	7.9	99	9.9
20	2.0	40	4.0	60	6.0	80	8.0	100	10.0

FLY MAGGOTS IN THE SKIN OF PETS

Maggots on or in skin wounds is a revolting thought, but it is a rather common finding, particularly in dogs. It can be seen in cats and dogs. This is caused by a pet having moist areas on the body or a skin wound that has been exposed to flies. Flies like to lay eggs in moist skin or open wounds. The eggs hatch, and maggots infest the moist skin or wounds. They are normally invasive in tissues and can be found at about any location on the body. Normally there are many, many maggots in any maggot infestation, and all have to be removed from the wound before starting any topical treatments.

TREATMENT
Maggots need to be removed and killed. Ivermectin will kill the maggots and can be given by injection under the skin, orally, or it can be placed directly onto the maggot infestation. (See Table 3.10 for dosages of Ivermectin.)

PREVENTION
Keeping the pet groomed and away from flies will prevent maggots from occurring on or in your pet.

Table 3.10 1 Percent Ivermectin Dose-by-Weight Chart

(weight divided by 80 = dose in cc)

Weight Pounds	Dose cc	Weight Pounds	Dose cc	Weight Pounds	Dose cc	Weight Pounds	Dose cc	Weight Pounds	Dose cc
1	0.01	21	0.26	41	0.51	61	0.76	81	1.01
2	0.02	22	0.27	42	0.52	62	0.77	82	1.02
3	0.03	23	0.28	43	0.53	63	0.78	83	1.03
4	0.05	24	0.30	44	0.55	64	0.80	84	1.05
5	0.06	25	0.31	45	0.56	65	0.81	85	1.06
6	0.07	26	0.32	46	0.57	66	0.82	86	1.07
7	0.08	27	0.33	47	0.58	67	0.83	87	1.08
8	0.10	28	0.35	48	0.60	68	0.85	88	1.10
9	0.11	29	0.36	49	0.61	69	0.86	89	1.11
10	0.12	30	0.37	50	0.62	70	0.87	90	1.12
11	0.13	31	0.38	51	0.63	71	0.88	91	1.13
12	0.15	32	0.40	52	0.65	72	0.90	92	1.15
13	0.16	33	0.41	53	0.66	73	0.91	93	1.16
14	0.17	34	0.42	54	0.67	74	0.92	94	1.17
15	0.18	35	0.43	55	0.68	75	0.93	95	1.18
16	0.20	36	0.45	56	0.70	76	0.95	96	1.20
17	0.21	37	0.46	57	0.71	77	0.96	97	1.21
18	0.22	38	0.47	58	0.72	78	0.97	98	1.22
19	0.23	39	0.49	59	0.73	79	0.98	99	1.23
20	0.25	40	0.50	60	0.75	80	1.00	100	1.25

EAR FLY BITES

Ear fly bites occur when a dog is in an area of filth that attracts flies. The tips of the ears may become raw from the bites of flies that land on the ears and cause open wounds, scabbing, and pain. If the dog has folded-over ears, the flies will bite at the area of the fold of the ear. Flies do not have biting parts, but they have burrs that are used to rub on the skin like a wire brush. This part of fly anatomy causes considerable trauma to the ears of pets.

If there are enough flies, the lesions normally seen on the ends of ears may also be seen on the face. When this occurs, the poor pet should be removed from the area where there are so many flies. Flies do not like dark areas; if any animal is pestered with flies, it can be placed in a dark area where the flies will not bother the animal. This can often be used on farms for cattle or horses that have problems with eye infections since flies are infamous for causing eye infections and skin wounds.

TREATMENT
Any triple antibiotic ointment that is available at grocery stores, pharmacies, or military PX or BX facilities can be used to treat the wounds of the ears. It is important that efforts be made to keep the pet out of reach of the flies. The dog should be kept from further exposure to flies until the ears are healed.

PREVENTION
Keep the dog out of areas where flies accumulate and multiply.

COCOON BY THE EYE (CUTEREBRA)

Actually it is not a cocoon, but it looks very much like a cocoon. Fly larvae are normally found in wild rabbits and rodents. The Cuterebra (pronounced cute-a-re-baa) fly tends to lay its eggs at the opening of rabbit and rodent burrows or runs. An indoor-outdoor cat is an investigator and needs to poke around. If the cat happens to poke its nose in the wrong place, it can become infected with the fly larvae of Cuterebra. The infection in cats seems more prevalent in summer months during fly season.

The cat will normally respond to the foreign body by creating an infection around the fly larvae. You may see indications associated with the infection caused by the larvae, such as red, inflamed skin around the embedded larvae. It is often found in the corner of the eye next to the nose, but it can be found at almost any location on the body. Most are found somewhere on the head. Cats sniff around, and the head is most often presented to the infective Cuterebra eggs first. Naturally, if the back happens to bump the egg nest, the larvae will be embedded somewhere on the cat's back.

When observing the wound, it will be noted that there are infectious materials around the larvae. If you look closely, you will see the larvae and an opening into the larvae with very small white spicules. The opening is necessary for survival of the larvae in the cat's body tissues. The goal is to remove the larvae without rupturing the larvae. The larvae are normally about half an inch or a centimeter long, about one-quarter inch or about 5 millimeters in diameter at the largest area.

TREATMENT

At times, anesthesia and minor surgery are required to remove the larvae; other times, gentle manipulating will allow removal. The pet's doctor most likely has seen this before and will be your best choice to do this for you.

PREVENTION

If allowed outdoors without supervision, there is little that can be done to prevent an accidental infection by the Cuterebra larvae.

DEMODEX EAR MITES

Occasionally demodex mites have been a cause of ear infestations in cats. Unlike the more common ear mites (*Otodectes cynotis*), these suckers are persistent and may require several weeks of treatment. Most owners do not have a microscope to look at ear contents.

If one should find persistent ear issues, which normally resolve with one or two treatments, consider one of two things that could be the reason: food allergies or demodex mites in the ears. A quick look into the ears will not distinguish between the common ear mites and demodex. Ears should be examined with an otoscope. Disposable plastic otoscopes are available for purchase at pharmacies such as CVS and Walgreens at reasonable prices. For diagnostic purposes, it will require looking at ear debris with a microscope to be able to see the demodex mites.

TREATMENT

Place about one half of a milliliter (cc) of Ivermectin in the ear and massage the ear well. It works well for treating the ear demodex mites. Treat daily for two weeks. Then stop and recheck at two and four weeks to make sure the ears are clear and clean. If you see black materials within the ear, you probably have not treated enough.

It may take a more persistent treatment plan to defeat the ear demodex infestation. If you suspect a food allergy, you need to change to a nonallergenic type of diet, which you can purchase at pet stores, such as Petco or PetSmart. It is easy for yeast infections to be in the ear; be aware of this possibility. Your pet's doctor may be able to help you determine the cause so you can proceed with good information and diagnosis.

PREVENTION

A routine checkup by you and your pet's doctor is the best you can do. When at the veterinary facility, you need to insist that they use an otoscope to look at your pet's ears. A quick look into the ear without an otoscope is not an adequate ear exam.

TAPEWORMS

Tapeworms are very common in dogs and cats. The infestation of the most common tapeworms that infect dogs and cats are the result of pets biting at and swallowing fleas that have eaten tapeworm eggs. Fleas on your pet will allow large numbers of tapeworms to be present in your pet's intestines.

I have seen such heavy infestations of tapeworms in cats that the poor cat vomits tapeworms. Adult tapeworms cause very little effect on the pet other than when the worm segments (proglottids) get stuck around the anus. These parts of tapeworms cause an itching sensation and may be a cause of scooting the back end on floors. This is a common sign with tapeworms, but I have never seen this to be true. Scooting on the floor has been found to be caused by impacted anal glands. I am sure some dude somewhere in this wide world has seen this—but not this dude. Signs of tapeworm infestation are not obvious unless the pet has a heavy infestation. The most common findings look like white rice (proglottids) on the feces when it is passed. This is often seen by owners and is the sign most often noted and reported.

The usual types of diagnostic techniques, such as fecal floatation, by your veterinarian may not be all that effective unless proglottids have expelled the tapeworm eggs. Most often, nothing is seen. The sight of white wiggly things on stool samples is the best way to identify tapeworms. One might see some parts of tapeworms around the anus of pets. However, most owners do not often look at the anus of their pet—so this is not an effective diagnostic way of determining if the pet has tapeworms. Stick with the little white wiggly things on stool samples.

The most common tapeworms are not normally a concern for infection in people. Young children who stick things in their mouths might accidentally be infected, and there are a few cases of people being infected with the common tapeworm. Most of these cases had special circumstances that set the stage for the infection. However, some tapeworms are very serious to humans if they happen to get infected with tapeworms. The *Echinococcus* tapeworms have had devastating effects in Australia.

Australia has no corner on the market when it comes to *Echinococcus* tapeworms. *Echinococcus* tapeworms in people can be really bad and can cause death. Other tapeworms can be caused by fecal-oral contamination or by eating partially cooked beef, lamb, and pork, which makes one who knows want well-cooked meats.

TREATMENT

If you have a preventive medicine program, you will probably never be bothered with tapeworms. However, if you do not, then the Panacur (Fenbendazole) chart below (Table 3.11) can be used to treat your pet. Obtain the dosage according to your pet's weight and give the medicine for three days. Repeat the treatment in two weeks and two weeks later to be sure.

PREVENTION

A good preventive medicine program is the best alternative. Making sure your pets have no fleas is a great way to prevent the most common tapeworms in dogs and cats. As with fleas, your pet will have tapeworms. Do you ever think of your cat or dog on your bed with fleas and tapeworms? Not a very comfortable thought, is it? Yuck.

Table 3.11 *Panacur (Fenbendazole) Dose-by-Weight Chart*

100 mg/cc Panacur [Fenbendazole] Dosing Chart
Repeat the dose for three days and then repeat
the three-day treatment in two weeks.
(weight times 25 divided by 100 = dose cc)

Weight Pounds	Dose cc	Weight Pounds	Dose cc	Weight Pounds	Dose cc	Weight Pounds	Dose cc	Weight Pounds	Dose cc
1	0.25	21	5.25	41	10.25	61	15.25	81	20.25
2	0.50	22	5.50	42	10.50	62	15.50	82	20.50
3	0.75	23	5.75	43	10.75	63	15.75	83	20.75
4	1.0	24	6.0	44	11.00	64	16.0	84	21.0
5	1.25	25	6.25	45	11.25	65	16.25	85	21.25
6	1.50	26	6.50	46	11.50	66	16.50	86	21.50
7	1.75	27	6.75	47	11.75	67	16.75	87	21.75
8	2.0	28	7.0	48	12.0	68	17.0	88	22.0
9	2.25	29	7.25	49	12.25	69	17.25	89	22.25
10	2.50	30	7.50	50	12.50	70	17.50	90	22.50
11	2.75	31	7.75	51	12.75	71	17.75	91	22.75
12	3.00	32	8.0	52	13.0	72	18.0	92	23.0
13	3.25	33	8.25	53	13.25	73	18.25	93	23.25
14	3.50	34	8.50	54	13.50	74	18.50	94	23.50
15	3.75	35	8.75	55	13.75	75	18.75	95	23.75
16	4.00	36	9.0	56	14.0	76	19.0	96	24.0
17	4.25	37	9.25	57	14.25	77	19.25	97	24.25
18	4.50	38	9.50	58	14.50	78	19.50	98	24.50
19	4.75	39	9.75	59	14.75	79	19.75	99	24.75
20	5.00	40	10.0	60	15.0	80	20.0	100	25.0

INSECT BITES

There are many insects that will bite or sting pets, including flies, bees, wasps, hornets, spiders, ants, mosquitoes. This discussion will focus on bees, wasps, spiders, and the common ant, black widow, and brown recluse spiders. These types of insects prefer warm weather and are more prevalent in the warm months of the year. It is during these periods that these insects are a menace to pets. Bites, depending upon the species, are more apt to occur on young, inquisitive animals. Cats may be a bit more tolerant to insect toxins than dogs are.

Stings from bees, wasps, hornets, and others most often occur without knowledge of the pet owner. The area may not be swollen, red, or sore. In many cases, the signs will depend on the location on the body, the number of times stung, and sensitivity to the venom being injected. Cats frequently get stung because they step on a nest of insects.

Mosquitoes like cats. Mosquitoes sting in areas that have less hair, such as the nose, the eye, and the ear. There may be redness and swelling at the sting site and often a lot of bite wounds noted. These mosquito stings can cause loss of hair at the sting wound site and often develop scabs or a crust at the locations of the stings on the ears and on the bridge of the nose. Improvement can be expected in four to seven days if one does not allow more mosquitoes to sting the cat.

Honeybees leave their stingers in the skin and have a barb on the end. The end sticking up may have a small swelling or an enlarged area close to the end of the stinger. This bulb has more venom in it; if squeezed, it will inject more venom into the pet. Remove this with caution so you do not inject more venom and cause more pain for the pet.

Wasps and hornets can sting multiple times and can have devastating effects on pets. If a pet happens to get a bee, wasp, or hornet in its mouth and is stung, the swelling and pain of the mouth may cause difficulty with breathing and death due to the swelling of tissues.

Local reactions are associated with immune responses that often include swelling of the face and generalized hives on the skin. A less common reaction is the development of anaphylaxis. Dog anaphylaxis signs may include vomiting, defecation, urination, muscular weakness, respiratory depression, or seizures. Cats with anaphylaxis may show an itching sensation, difficulty breathing, salivation, incoordination, or collapsing.

Black widow stings can result in mild to severe systemic signs that may include muscle pain, weakness, paralysis, and death. Cats are very sensitive to black widow venom and have death rates of up to 90 percent. Very young and old animals may be more sensitive to black widow venom. Physical findings might include vomiting, muscle pain, rigidity, tremors, cramping, and rapid breathing.

Brown recluse spider bites are not as common as other insect bites. Brown recluse stings on animals are rather rare. This is partly due to the limited areas of the country where the spiders are found. Signs of a sting from a brown recluse include pain, itching, and redness of the skin, which can be seen normally within ten to thirty minutes. The recluse causes a "bull's-eye" or "halo" skin lesion that progressively expands, and there may be central exudates (pus) vesicles that may rupture and become shrunken. These are dark purple or black. Skin lesions can be rather small, about a half-inch (one centimeter) in diameter or larger than nine inches (twenty-five centimeters) in diameter, and are not necessarily round. The size depends on how long the bite has been present.

Ants tend to bite pets on the underside of the body and can cause pain due to multiple bite wounds. Often the bites are in circular patterns. In time, the bites can turn black.

TREATMENT

The first issue is to actually identify the signs of a sting wound since they often occur without knowledge of the owner. Treatment can include cold packs, application of triple antibiotic ointments that contain local anesthetic compound, and Benadryl at one (1) milligram per pound (two [2] milligrams per kilogram) to two (2) milligrams per pound (four [4] milligrams per kilogram) of body weight.

PREVENTION

This is a difficult problem to prevent. Black widows may be found near a pool, an outhouse, on a farm, or near trash. If you happen to know of such areas, they can be treated to eliminate the spiders. Others are chance occurrences—just as a mosquito may bite you on the arm.

Table 3.12 *Benadryl Dog and Cat Dose-by-Weight Chart*

25 mg tablets are available OTC. Dosage is based on cut
25 mg tablets, which cannot be precisely accurate.
Remember dose is close—not accurate due to cut tablets.

Weight Pounds	Dose # Tablets and/or Tablet Parts	Weight Pounds	Dose # Tablets and/or Tablet Parts	Weight Pounds	Dose # Tablets and/or Tablet Parts	Weight Pounds	Dose # Tablets and/or Tablet Parts	Weight Pounds	Dose # Tablets and/or Tablet Parts
1	1/8=.12	21	1.75	41	3.25	61	5	81	6.50
2	¼= .25	22	1.75	42	3.25	62	5	82	6.50
3	¼=.25	23	1.75	43	3.50	63	5	83	6.75
4	½+¼ =3/4 =.75	24	2	44	3.50	64	5.12	84	6.75
5	½=.50	25	2	45	3.75	65	5.25	85	6.75
6	½=.50	26	2	46	3.75	66	5.25	86	6
7	½=.50	27	2.12	47	3.75	67	5.25	87	6.75+.12
8	.50+.12	28	2.25	48	3.75	68	5.50	88	7
9	.50+.25	29	2.25	49	3.75+.12	69	5.50	89	7
10	.50+.25	30	2.50	50	4	70	5.50	90	7.25
11	1	31	2.50	51	4	71	5.75	91	7.25
12	1	32	2.50	52	4.12	72	5.75	92	7.25
13	1	33	2.75	53	4.25	73	5.75	93	7.50
14	1.12	34	2.75	54	4.25	74	6	94	7.50
15	1.25	35	2.75	55	4.50	75	6	95	7.50
16	1.25	36	2.75+.12	56	4.50	76	6	96	7.75
17	1.25	37	3	57	4.50	77	6.12	97	7.75
18	1.50	38	3	58	4.50	78	6.25	98	8
19	1.50	39	3.12	59	4.75	79	6.25	99	8
20	1.50+.12	40	3.25	60	4.75	80	6.50	100	8

1/8 = .12 tablet, ¼ = .25 tablet, ½ = .5 tablet, ½ + ¼ = ¾ = .75 tablet

INTERNAL PARASITES

Internal parasites are one of the most common health issues for cats and dogs, and they are easy to treat and prevent if an owner knows what to do to treat or prevent these diseases. Parasites have such intricate life cycles that it seems like it would be impossible for them to be so successful at infecting animals and people. Parasites have been around for thousands of years and are very efficient at surviving and infecting animals.

The two most common parasites in dogs and cats are hookworms and roundworms. These two parasites can be obtained directly from the mother to the young at birth by nursing or direct infections. Newborn dogs can have the parasites in their intestines at birth and have positive fecal exams at one week of age. Hookworms can penetrate the skin. Hookworms and roundworms can be obtained by fecal-oral contamination or by eating a small animal that is infected with parasites. Hookworms and roundworms can cause parasitic infections in humans.

Hookworms are bloodsucking parasites that cause anemia in dogs and cats. It has been calculated that one hookworm can remove about 0.8 cc or milliliter in twenty-four hours (E. J. L. Soulsby, *Helminths, Arthropods, and Protozoa of Domesticated Animals*, 6th edition, p. 216). That is close to one milliliter in twenty-four hours. A hundred worms will drink a lot of blood very fast. It is no wonder that hookworms will make a pet acquire iron deficiency anemia very quickly or kill the pet due to loss of blood. Like many parasites, hookworms can penetrate the skin, complete a systemic migration through the body, and end up in the intestines.

Roundworms infect cats and dogs by fecal-oral ingestion and can infect people. Depending on the type, a roundworm may migrate and cause visceral (abdominal) and/or eye migration. It has been said (I have not seen this sign in any pets) that roundworms can cause hiccups in pets. Roundworms can also be vomited if the infection is heavy.

Whipworms are primarily found in dogs but can also infect cats. Tapeworms are common in cats, and most are acquired by biting at and swallowing fleas. The more fleas a cat swallows, the more tapeworms it can have. Cats can be so full of tapeworms that they vomit them.

TREATMENT

There are many treatments for parasites. De-wormers are available at pet stores or 1 (800) Pet-Meds. Follow directions on the package. Panacur is a good wormer for all of the above parasites. Panacur can be also be purchased at pet stores and feed stores. If purchased at a feed store, buy 100 mg/cc Panacur.

Table 3.13 can be used to obtain the dose for the 100 mg/cc Panacur obtained at feed stores. Treat with Panacur for three days and repeat the three-day treatment in two weeks. If you treat your pet with Revolution, it will treat roundworms and hookworms—but not whipworms or tapeworms. Praziquantel or Praziquantel with Pyrantel Pamoate (Drontal or Droncit) will also treat tapeworms and is available at pet stores, online, and at 1 (800) PetMeds. Ivermectin will also treat hookworms, roundworms, and whipworms.

Special Note: When treating intestinal parasites, the only worms treated are those in the intestines at the time of treatment. Hookworms and roundworms have migration phases; if the worms are in migration, they are not treated. So treat once—and two weeks later, treat again. Two weeks later, have a stool sample checked. Or treat a third time and then have a stool sample checked. If the pet has a negative stool sample, recheck a stool sample one month later just to be sure it is still negative. This will make you feel comfortable that you have cleaned out the parasites.

Table 3.13 *Panacur (Fenbendazole) Dose-by-Weight Chart*

100 mg/Cc Panacur [Fenbendazole] Dosing Chart
Repeat the dose for three days and then repeat
the three-day treatment in two weeks.
(weight times 25 divided by 100 = dose by cc)

Weight Pounds	Dose cc	Weight Pounds	Dose cc	Weight Pounds	Dose cc	Weight Pounds	Dose cc	Weight Pounds	Dose cc
1	0.25	21	5.25	41	10.25	61	15.25	81	20.25
2	0.50	22	5.50	42	10.50	62	15.50	82	20.50
3	0.75	23	5.75	43	10.75	63	15.75	83	20.75
4	1.0	24	6.0	44	11.00	64	16.0	84	21.0
5	1.25	25	6.25	45	11.25	65	16.25	85	21.25
6	1.50	26	6.50	46	11.50	66	16.50	86	21.50
7	1.75	27	6.75	47	11.75	67	16.75	87	21.75
8	2.0	28	7.0	48	12.0	68	17.0	88	22.0
9	2.25	29	7.25	49	12.25	69	17.25	89	22.25
10	2.50	30	7.50	50	12.50	70	17.50	90	22.50
11	2.75	31	7.75	51	12.75	71	17.75	91	22.75
12	3.00	32	8.0	52	13.0	72	18.0	92	23.0
13	3.25	33	8.25	53	13.25	73	18.25	93	23.25
14	3.50	34	8.50	54	13.50	74	18.50	94	23.50
15	3.75	35	8.75	55	13.75	75	18.75	95	23.75
16	4.00	36	9.0	56	14.0	76	19.0	96	24.0
17	4.25	37	9.25	57	14.25	77	19.25	97	24.25
18	4.50	38	9.50	58	14.50	78	19.50	98	24.50
19	4.75	39	9.75	59	14.75	79	19.75	99	24.75
20	5.00	40	10.0	60	15.0	80	20.0	100	25.0

THREADWORMS (STRONGYLE) INTESTINAL INFECTION

Strongyloides are parasites that will infect people and animals in a heartbeat and cause profuse diarrhea. It is interesting that the parasitic form of this parasite is all-female parasites. This parasite is the reason the fecal samples need to be fresh to make a correct diagnosis. An old fecal specimen can have hookworms in it—and with time will look like the parasite of *Strongyloides stercoralis*. This parasite will self-infect a person or pet within the intestinal tract as well as penetrate skin and migrate until it gets into the intestinal tract.

This parasite infects dog, cats, people, monkeys, and a host of other animals. It is a very persistent, and it is hard to completely resolve the parasite issue. When it comes to parasite challenges, this will test one's persistence and consistency.

This parasite is one that puppies can get in the milk of the mother, and it will kill the puppies in a very short period of time. If the parasites penetrate the skin, the pet will experience a period of feeling the need to scratch at the skin where the parasites penetrated. At the time of the itching, there are no other signs—and one wonders why the scratching is occurring. This occurs in people if they get the parasite through the skin. The parasite will also penetrate through clothes.

Fecal-oral contamination is another way of obtaining the parasite. The parasites migrate through the lungs—depending upon the numbers—and can create a lung infection. Infections of skin and lungs are present before the intestinal phenomenon occurs.

TREATMENT

If your pet has this parasite, it is not a treat for three or four days and treatment must continue until multiple negative fecal tests are competed as late as 3 months after treatment stops. I have seen some treatment plans that gave medications only until the diarrhea was under control. This type of treatment plan does not cure or eliminate the parasite. Treatment only kills those parasites that are in the intestines.

If the treatment period is only until the diarrhea is under control, it will come back in full force. The parasite will penetrate the intestines and perianal area and reinfect the patient. To treat the parasite, one has to treat constantly and persistently for three or four months. To be sure, it may take longer to kill the parasite and rid the pet of the parasites.

Different products can be used for treatment. Panacur can be used constantly for several months, but the best choice may be Ivermectin. With Ivermectin, the *Merck Manual* states that a second treatment may be necessary. Treatment must continue until *multiple* fecal tests are negative. You must be persistent for successful treatment of this parasite. Do not give up. Hang in there until your pet is free of Strongyloides. Panacur can be purchased at pet stores, such as PetSmart and Petco, and at feed stores. If you purchase Panacur (Fenbendazole) at pet stores, follow the directions on the package. If you purchase Panacur (Fenbendazole) at feed stores, be sure to purchase 100 mg per cc and use the dosage chart below according to your pet's weigh. Do not overdose your pet; use the correct dose according to your pet's weight. (See Table 3.14.)

PREVENTION

Good sanitation involves staying out of areas where parasites may be obtained, such as dog parks. From personal experience, if you ever have a reason to be in an area that has monkeys overhead, do not sit down—and do not allow your pets into these areas. Monkeys defecate, and the grounds and surrounding areas will be contaminated with this parasite. (This has occurred in the Panama Canal area.)

Table 3.14 *Panacur (Fenbendazole) Dose-by-Weight Chart*

100 mg/cc Panacur [Fenbendazole] Dosing Chart
Repeat the dose for three days and then repeat
the three-day treatment in two weeks.
(weight times 25 divided by 100 = dose by cc)

Weight Pounds	Dose cc	Weight Pounds	Dose cc	Weight Pounds	Dose cc	Weight Pounds	Dose cc	Weight Pounds	Dose cc
1	0.25	21	5.25	41	10.25	61	15.25	81	20.25
2	0.50	22	5.50	42	10.50	62	15.50	82	20.50
3	0.75	23	5.75	43	10.75	63	15.75	83	20.75
4	1.0	24	6.0	44	11.00	64	16.0	84	21.0
5	1.25	25	6.25	45	11.25	65	16.25	85	21.25
6	1.50	26	6.50	46	11.50	66	16.50	86	21.50
7	1.75	27	6.75	47	11.75	67	16.75	87	21.75
8	2.0	28	7.0	48	12.0	68	17.0	88	22.0
9	2.25	29	7.25	49	12.25	69	17.25	89	22.25
10	2.50	30	7.50	50	12.50	70	17.50	90	22.50
11	2.75	31	7.75	51	12.75	71	17.75	91	22.75
12	3.00	32	8.0	52	13.0	72	18.0	92	23.0
13	3.25	33	8.25	53	13.25	73	18.25	93	23.25
14	3.50	34	8.50	54	13.50	74	18.50	94	23.50
15	3.75	35	8.75	55	13.75	75	18.75	95	23.75
16	4.00	36	9.0	56	14.0	76	19.0	96	24.0
17	4.25	37	9.25	57	14.25	77	19.25	97	24.25
18	4.50	38	9.50	58	14.50	78	19.50	98	24.50
19	4.75	39	9.75	59	14.75	79	19.75	99	24.75
20	5.00	40	10.0	60	15.0	80	20.0	100	25.0

CHAPTER 4

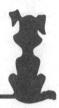

NUTRITION AND EATING PROBLEMS

It's a funny thing about life. If you refuse to accept
everything but the best, you very often get it.
—W. Somerset Maugham

Nutrition is a very essential part of good health for any animal. It is important that all necessary nutrients and vitamins are in the diets of dogs and cats.

Feeding free choice often results in overweight pets. It is not the free choice that is the problem. The problem is the amount of food in the free-choice container for the pets. Too much is too much. Leaving excess food down for days on end is not good. Pets like fresh foods and shun old foods.

It does not take a rocket scientist to know that dogs and cats will tire of their foods, and a variety of foodstuffs seems to encourage normal food consumption. The biggest issue is that a pet, unlike a person, cannot bebop over to the refrigerator and make another sandwich. So limiting the food is good when it comes to weight control. Hiding food from cats in puzzle balls has been of benefit for some cats in that they have to hunt and somewhat forage for food.

Dogs and cats have different nutritional needs. As an example of nutritional needs, when we went to Malaysia, we had to quarantine our cat for ninety days—and they fed dog food to the cats. When we could pick her up, we noticed she had a new mixture of white hairs on her body, and it took months for normal hair to come back. In this chapter, we will discuss a variety of issues as they relate to pet nutrients, some directly and some indirectly. Remember a well-fed pet is normally a healthy pet.

KEEPING MY PET'S WEIGHT CORRECT

"He is not fat—he's just fluffy!" Pet owners are often late to recognize that their pets may be overweight or underweight. We tend to take the easy road and feed free choice or have food available 24–7, and it turns out to be absolutely the wrong thing to do. The issue is identifying the appropriate feeding protocol or best methods for our pet. This is a challenge for pet weight control—and for pet owners. However, it is the key to controlling our pet's weight and preventing obesity or emaciation.

According to a recent survey by the Association for Pet Obesity Prevention, 53 percent of our nation's adult dogs and 55 percent of our cats are overweight. That amounts to 88.4 million overweight pets in the USA. There has to be a simple way to determine if a pet is in the correct weight zone. There is a simple way to determine if your pet's weight is within the proper range—and you can make adjustments to the daily amounts.

Here is how you can make a difference in your pet's weight and ensure that your pet's weight is within the proper weight range:

1. Run your fingertips over your pet's ribs against the direction of the animal's hair coat, without applying pressure. If you feel your pet's ribs, the pet is most likely underweight.
2. If you can't feel your pet's ribs, rub your fingers in the direction of the hair coat, but this time, apply light pressure against the ribs. If you feel the ribs easily, your animal is at a healthy weight.
3. If there is a layer of fat covering the animal's ribs, this is an indication that the pet is obese.

One needs to manage a pet's weight because overweight pets can have other health issues. The disease that is most common due to excessive weight is diabetes, and we do not want to be pumping insulin into our pets. We need to keep the weight down.

Excess food down is the method of feeding that allows pets to help themselves. This is the perfect way to cause your pet to gain weight. It is an almost guaranteed way for weight gain in pets. The solution is to feed smaller amounts. I personally make sure that the bottom of the dish used to feed our pets can be easily seen. Reduction of the amount of food you are feeding is essential for helping maintain a pet's weight. Be careful not to create underweight pets. Keep an eye out or weigh your pet after a period of time on the lower amount of food being fed.

There is always a chance that your pet has some undetectable disease, such as hypothyroid, low thyroid levels, or hormonal issues that only the pet's doctor can detect with blood tests. Obviously any unnoticed systemic disease needs to be ruled out so you do not find yourself banging your head against the wall.

Some owner behavior modification becomes necessary. A successful pet weight-management program will require permanent changes to your pet-feeding behavior. For example, you need to limit treats. Pay attention to calories, carbohydrates, and fat content of pet food and treats.

PREVENTION

Weight control in pets is a real challenge for pet owners—just as it is for people. Many of the same things involved in weight of people apply to pets. There are some specific things we can do to help our pet's weight. We can remove the pet from the dining room when eating meals. We can limit treats and make sure the treats are not fattening. Ideally all foods—including treats—should be put in the pet's feeding bowl only. Finally, we can provide attention and rewards that do not involve food.

ALL-MEAT DIETS

To start this discussion, it needs to be said that no animal should be fed an all-meat diet. The source of the meat is not the issue. It makes no difference if it is chicken, turkey, or large-animal muscle meats, such as buffalo or beef. The striated muscle meats (muscle meats) of animals can bring on issues caused by an all-meat diet. In the professional world, this would be called *nutritional secondary hyperparathyroidism* or *pseudo hyperparathyroidism.*

The all-meat syndrome is due to calcium and phosphorus levels that the body needs to maintain a normal equilibrium and stay healthy. Normal blood calcium and phosphorus level should have a ratio of plus or minus 1.1 through 2.2 calcium to 1 phosphorus. When an all-striated muscle meat diet is fed, phosphorus levels in the muscle meat become very high. This causes the level of calcium to phosphorus to change in the body to a high phosphorus level and a ratio of perhaps one or two calcium to twelve or fifteen phosphorus or higher.

The body is a marvelous organism that does all it can to protect and prevent damage to itself and attempts to heal itself. In the case of the all-meat diets, the body needs to maintain body blood levels of calcium to phosphorus ratios. Due to the lack of calcium in muscle meats, the consumer of the diet has to recruit calcium from somewhere else to maintain body equilibrium. The body receives a signal through the endocrine systems that calcium is needed in the circulating bloodstream. The only source of calcium in the body is from the bones.

The body recruits calcium from bones, causing the bones to become much thinner over time due to the abundance of calcium. The bones will become thin, unable to support the animal's weight, and the bones will start to crumble, fold, and break. The dog may develop dandruff and/or diarrhea. It is hard to understand why a dog has a broken leg or diarrhea. It seems hard to understand what has happened to the pet. The owner might think they have been giving their pet the best diet available, but they are killing their pet.

This syndrome has been scientifically documented, and the results were published in professional journals. (*American Veterinary Medical Association Journal*, February 15, 1971) At one time, there was a diet on the market that caused this syndrome in many, many dogs. Now it occurs not due to a known commercial diet on the available market— but by owners who feed all-meat diets from homemade meals.

I have seen this syndrome in a small dog that was only fed chicken and turkey meat. The jaw was broken, and radiographs showed the bones were very thin. The bones were so thin that trying to repair the fracture would have caused considerable more damage to the bone; therefore, the jaw fracture could not be fixed.

Another time, I was visiting with a veterinarian and was asked to view a radiograph of a fracture. The first observation noted how thin the bones were. The owner happened to be in the lobby. A discussion with the owner revealed the pet was being fed an all-meat diet with green beans. The owner was shocked to learn the diet was creating such a problem in her dog. The fact that some vegetables were being fed may have slowed the bone absorption somewhat, but it never stopped it. After explaining the problem, the owner said she would change the diet.

TREATMENT

The best treatment is simply not to feed any animal an all-meat diet. A little meat occasionally is not the same as an all-meat diet. I recommend a good commercial diet. I personally feed Science Diet brands, which is a well-balanced diet that is scientifically designed for cats and dogs.

PREVENTION

Do not feed an all-meat diet to pets.

SENSITIVE STOMACH OF CATS

When feeding cats, many folks tend to put lots of food in a bowl so they do not have to feed frequently. This is not a good practice for many reasons. Some difficulties that stem from a bottomless food bowl include weight gain, diabetes, and stimulation for vomiting in some cats.

Two things will stimulate nonpersistent vomiting in housecats. It probably occurs in feral cats, but it has not been observed. The two stimuli are eating plants and overeating. The cat will normally vomit plant material a short time after consuming it. The cat seems to wait until it is back in the house and on the rug to begin vomiting. The cat is not sick, but the plant materials act as a limited cause of emesis or vomiting, making a mess.

Excess food will act as a nonpersistent emetic, causing the cat to vomit. Frequently the food is still formed in its original kibble shape—with some fluids—and occasionally even some plant materials. As the food is discharged from the cat, it may be formed in the shape of a tube due to the esophagus being a round pipe—or the cat's vomit can be an amorphous mess with food and liquid. If not found right away, it seems to dry. The cat is not sick and normally goes on its merry way as though nothing has happened.

It is important to know that the vomiting is due to overeating or eating small amounts of plant materials. The general condition of the cat is normal. The cat will eat and play normally, and all other activities are normal. It is important that the vomiting is not persistent.

Some vomitus will be a liquid that looks colorless or yellow. The yellow color means the fluid is coming from the duodenum and not the stomach. The duodenum is the part of the intestines that the stomach contents and bile are excreted into. The bile causes the yellow color.

A colorless or yellow fluid seen only once and not repeated is not a reason to see the pet's doctor. At our facility, we see this every once in a while, and we have not determined why it happens—but it does. However, persistent vomiting can be very serious, and one should take the pet to see the pet's doctor since it could be due to a foreign body blockage or systemic condition that needs professional help.

If the vomitus looks like black coffee grounds, it normally means the pet is vomiting blood from some unknown cause.

TREATMENT

There is no treatment for a nonpersistent vomiting cat. The treatment in this case is to limit plants available to the cat and to lower the amount of foods you offer and put into the feeding bowl. In my case, the cat at our house has this syndrome. We often feed Greenies treats; if the cat is given more than five treats at a time, it is almost a guarantee that the cat will vomit soon. It is seldom on easy-to-clean areas, but it does occur sometimes.

PREVENTION

Prevention for this is about the same as the treatment with this particular syndrome. Remember to limit plants in and around the house—and do not put too much food in the food bowls. Determining how much food to feed your pet may be similar to a titration you may have done in chemistry class in high school or college. You just give the amount that the cat will eat that does not stimulate vomiting. You will have no mess to clean up.

MY CAT STOPPED EATING

Cats that refuse to eat seem to be rather common. In most cases, there are underlying diseases that make the cat feel badly. The problem in almost all cases is beyond the ability of home diagnosis and treatment. Many things could be provoking this dilemma, including cancer, diabetes, upper respiratory infections, and dehydration. Other conditions that might be a stimulus for not eating are a change in diets, separation from the owner (e.g., boarding), harassment by another pet, a new puppy, or a dominant cat.

Dehydration is associated with not eating and can be quite severe. When a cat stops eating, it is predisposed to *fatty liver syndrome*. If a cat has not eaten for about seven days, the liver starts to become infiltrated with natural fats and triglycerides. Normally, 80 percent of the liver is at risk. Overweight cats are a bit more prone to development of this condition.

The syndrome is not understood very well, but fatty liver

syndrome can result in death of the cat. It is a challenge to treat. A cat must get nutrition to reverse the development of the fatty liver problem—and the underlying cause that made the cat stop eating. Failure to eat makes this a very complex disease for cats. Other signs to watch for include lethargy, weight loss, yellow skin—or yellowing of the whites of the eyes—and persistent, recurring vomiting.

TREATMENT

Unfortunately, this issue is definitely a challenge for the pet's doctor to overcome due to the complexity of the issues that may be involved in the development of the fatty liver syndrome. The most important thing is getting the cat to eat. This can be done by force feeding or using an oral gastric feeding tube to get food into the cat's stomach. The problem with a vomiting cat is keeping the food down. The cat's doctor will have the resources to diagnose and treat the many types of issues that may be identified—if they are treatable.

PREVENTION

It is difficult to predict if the cat will ever develop the syndrome of not eating, and there is no specific program that can be followed to ensure the cat will continue to eat. The best prevention is to be aware of a cat not eating and not wait seven days to allow a fatty liver to develop. Take your cat to see the veterinarian right away; the sooner the problem is overcome, the better the survival rates will be.

STOMACH DILATATION OR BLOAT

Bloat is a condition in which a dog's stomach fills partially with air and partially with water. This is a condition that can occur quickly and can occur when a large dog is being prepared for surgery. We have seen this in surgery. The stomach starts to fill rapidly with air, and the stomach can be observed expanding quickly. It started to be such a common occurrence that we kept a tube to run down the esophagus to let the air out of the stomach. This strange occurrence seemed to happen frequently with no identifiable cause. The good news is that it has not occurred for a long time at our facility.

Many things can be the cause of bloat. Large dogs that have had anesthesia for surgery and go home on the same day should have limited access to water. I believe in limiting water until the next day. Cases of bloat in large dogs have occurred after surgery. In each case, an owner allowed a pet to drink all the water it wanted. Do not allow a postsurgery dog to have lots of water. It seems to be a trigger for bloat, especially in larger dogs. When bloat happens, it comes on fast—and it is an emergency if the dog has to be saved. Surgery has to be done that evening or afternoon—or as soon as it is recognized. If recognized late, the doctor may not be able to save the pet.

Bloat likes large dogs, and it is seen on hot days when dogs have been worked or run hard. When they return home, they tend to drink a lot of water, which may be a trigger for expansion and twisting of the stomach on its long axis. When the stomach twists, a tube cannot be inserted through the esophagus to the stomach due to the blockage of the esophagus caused by the stomach twisting and creating blockage of the esophagus and the intestines at the other end of the stomach.

This combination of a dilated stomach, twisted tissues, and stoppage of blood flow to the tissues involved creates an immediate emergency situation for several reasons. The stomach will have twisted on the long axis—between halfway and completely blocking entry and exit from the stomach. The stomach will start to expand (bloat) and cause increased pressure against the diaphragm, which impacts the lungs, causing breathing issues on top of all the other things that are happening. The twisted tissues cause blood circulation problems that lead to shock and death.

Signs you may see in a case of bloat include trying to vomit but nothing comes up, distended abdomen that feels hard, strings of saliva hanging from the mouth, and the appearance of pain. If no one is around when this happens, the dog may be found on the floor and will not respond to any sounds.

TREATMENT

If the dog is to survive, emergency surgery is required as soon as possible. Delay may mean death.

PREVENTION

In my personal experience, it seems that giving excessive water to a dog after being out in the heat causes bloat in dogs. Therefore, when finished with activities outside on hot days, do not give free choice water. Other causative events are in the twilight zone and are not known.

Unfortunately, no preventive direction can be given. However, when bloat starts to occur, the abdomen starts to expand. The abdomen seems to get large rather fast. If you see this happening, it is time to head to the pet's emergency doctor.

CONTAMINATED PET FOODS

It is unfortunate that commercial foods sometimes become contaminated with organisms that cause them to be recalled. The most common bacteria in pet food is the *salmonella* species. There are other organisms that contaminate pet foods.

Salmonella seems to be the most frequent contaminate found in pet foods in the United States, but this is reported to be a rare occurrence. There are online sites you can use to look up pet foods to see if the pet food has been recalled. The American Veterinary Medical Association provides a site that is maintained frequently. You can view this site online at www.avma.org/News/Issues/recalls-alerts. The US Food and Drug Administration also has a site at www.fda.gov/AnimalVeterinary/SafetyHealth/RecallsWithdrawals. In addition, the Centers for Disease Control and Prevention has a site that provides tips for handling pet food safely, which can be found online at www.cdc.gov/Features/SalmonellaDryPetFood. The good news is that contamination of pet foods has been on the decline, but salmonella remains the leading cause of pet-food recalls.

One of the most common sources of salmonella contamination happens to be found in so-called raw food products. Raw diets consist of food products, such as pig's ears, jerky treats, eggs, poultry, milk, and meat that have not been cooked or treated for elimination of bacteria. These food items are most commonly found to be the sources of contamination of bacteria and are most harmful to pets and people.

The contamination of pet food as a source of illness for pets turns out to be uncommon. The more common issue is that the pet becomes an infected carrier of the food contaminant bacteria. Salmonella is a source of infection and illness in family members. The family members most susceptible to this type of exposure are under the age of five, older than sixty-five, and those with compromised immune systems. This does not necessarily exempt other members of the family from becoming infected.

Here are some tips to help protect you and your family from such an illness. When purchasing dry pet foods, look at the bag to make sure there are no visible signs of damage to the package, such as tears, discoloration, or water damage, which might contaminate the contents of the bag. Avoid purchasing damaged canned foods. A small dent in a can be a source of very small holes in the can that allow contamination. Remember that bacteria are microscopic in size and can enter the smallest openings possible.

Above all, avoid raw diets for your pets. It is important to reiterate that raw products are the top source of pet-food illness in pets and family members. The CDC recommends against feeding raw food products to dogs or cats due to the possibility of illness. It has been determined that is it is best to wash one's hands with soap and water for at least twenty seconds after handling pet food treats—and especially before preparing or serving food and drinks to family members or preparing baby bottles.

Pet foods can be a source of bacterial contamination, and some tips about storage of pet foods that may be beneficial. If possible, store dry pet foods in original bags inside a clean plastic container with a lid. Store in a dry area with a temperature lower than eighty degrees (26.6 Celsius). Properly refrigerate or discard unused, leftover, wet pet food and containers. Washing hands is recommended by CDC after handling dry dog food due to potential bacterial contamination.

As most parents know, toddlers like to place things in their mouths. Allowing a young child around a pet's food bowl—or into a dry pet food bag—may be a source of bacterial illness for a young child. Every effort should be made to keep youngsters from obtaining pet foods to prevent unwanted illnesses.

Pet food manufacturers are making major efforts to prevent bacterial and salmonella contamination in pet foods at every phase of the manufacturing processes. While pet-food recalls seem to get lots of attention, they are uncommon, and most customers are satisfied with their pet food products.

HAIRBALLS IN CATS

Hairballs (trichobezoars) are a constant problem in cats due to their grooming habits, and they can be more of an issue in long-haired cats than in short-haired cats. Hairballs can cause vomiting, and if there happen to be underlying conditions, there is always the possibility of more difficult intestinal issues. Hairballs are frequently related to intestinal problems and/or skin-hair-coat problems or associated neurological diseases. If there are other cats in the household, it is possible that a cat will groom the other cats too. These issues may complicate hairball problems.

In the normal cat, hairballs might stimulate occasional vomiting. Some cats will not eat much for one or two days after discharging the hairballs. If this persists beyond two days, it is best to see your pet's doctor to ensure that there no other issues. Waiting beyond this time may be detrimental to the health of your cat. Pay attention to your cat's hairball issue. It is wise to be proactive rather than sorry. If you are familiar with the cat's past actions, you will probably be more attuned to the needs of your cat.

TREATMENT

This treatment is for noncomplicated cases of hairballs. At most grocery stores, you can purchase Carnation or Pet condensed/evaporated milk and feed it to your cat. Do not dilute the condensed milk by adding anything to it. Serve it as it comes in the can. The concentration of the milk will remove hairballs. Normally this will clean the cat within a few hours.

There are other treatments you can use that require smearing ointments or ointment-like products on the feet of your cat. The ointments are then cleaned off by the cat, which treats hairballs. This includes Vaseline and other products for hairballs that are available at pet stores such as PetSmart or Petco. These later treatments have a downside in that the cat may get these products onto furniture and rugs.

PREVENTION

As cats tend to groom themselves frequently, it is difficult—if not impossible—to prevent hairballs. However, one can schedule a routine hairball treatment with condensed milk. It is simple. Just allow the cat to have the condensed milk every two weeks, once a month, or every two months as you see the need. This will prevent large accumulations of hairballs.

BAD BREATH (HALITOSIS)

There are numerous things that cause bad breath in cats and dogs. A large percentage of oral smells can be due to dirty teeth, oral infections of the gums due to dirty teeth, or from eating feces and other foul-smelling foods or food wastes.

Many people are using pet toothbrushes to combat bad breath and to improve the oral health of their pets. Many grocery stores now have disposable dental teeth scrapes and picks that can be used on pet teeth. One never knows what can be done with a pet's teeth without the use of anesthesia until one tries to scrape a dirty tooth. You will be surprised by what your pet may allow you to do.

Recently our clinic had a cat with excessive accumulation of food and other products on its back molars. We were able to completely clean the teeth easily with a tooth scraper. If we had used anesthesia and completed blood tests, it would have cost a minimum of $200. We tried scraping—and we did it in within minutes at no cost. The next animal may not allow us to do the same thing, but it is worth giving it a shot with your pet. To paraphrase an insurance advertisement, you could save a lot of money if you switch to trying.

If a dog has a habit of eating feces, the best treatment is to pick up the feces as soon as it is produced. It is the best prevention. There is no other process that will work as well. It takes a little effort, but it certainly stops the eating of feces.

Soft foods tend to accumulate quickly on teeth of pets, and it is this accumulation that adds to bad breath. It creates bad teeth and causes gum infections. Hard, dry foods tend to pop off or help remove accumulations on the teeth.

Just to clarify: I did not say hard food cleans the teeth. I said it helps to clean the teeth—and dry foods actually help to improve bad breath.

TREATMENT

Brushing teeth works wonders for pet breath and oral health. Not all animals will be happy to allow you to brush their teeth, but many will—so give it a try. SV Distribution has an online product called ProDen PlaqueOff™, which can be purchased at www.svdist.com (formally www.international-dental.com). This product can be used in dogs and cats and will help bad breath and oral health. SV Distribution's telephone number is 909-646-9949. ProDen PlaqueOff™ is a bit expensive, but if directions are followed, it will last about a year, making it a rather cost-effective product. It can be purchased in different sizes to best fit your needs.

There are other products that help bad breath. Tartar Shield is available online at www.tartarshield.com. It is a food-like product and is effective if used. Tartar Shield's telephone number is 317-565-7658 and their free telephone number is 888-598-7658. PetSmart and Petco have several products that can help with bad breath and oral health.

PREVENTION

A good oral-health plan will do wonders for preventing bad breath. Good oral health has been shown to extend the life of many pets.

Yours can be among the long-lived pets if you make the effort to have your pet among those with good oral health.

INTESTINAL GAS (FLATULENCE)

Gas passing is more problematic in dogs than in cats, and it can be an issue. The gases that are passed are normally the result of three major sources. Gas is present in the gut as the result of swallowed air, diet, or the diffusion of gas into the intestines from blood.

The amount of gas diffused from blood is normally insignificant. If blood gas diffusion does occur, the gas diffused into the gut is almost all nitrogen. The largest producer of intestinal gas or flatulence is due to digestion byproducts in the intestines. Almost no intestinal gas originates from swallowed air or blood gas diffusion.

Bacterial metabolism in the intestinal tract produces significant volumes of hydrogen, methane, and carbon dioxide. Diet accounts for majority of the flatus production in dogs, and differences in the colonic flora and motility may have an influence on the gas production. If the dog has not been having a problem—and it comes on all of a sudden—it could be due to a bacteria overgrowth. If so, you will need help from the pet's doctor.

When people swallow air, it results more in belching than in flatus—and it is assumed to be about the same in dogs.

TREATMENT

Three approaches can be taken to diminish gas passing in dogs. Since the major portion of intestinal gas is due to bacterial actions on the contents of the intestines, different diets may be the best answer. One has to try different types of diets to hit upon the one that is best for the pet.

A low-fiber diet might not work in all dogs, but it's a starting point. Gas X (smethicone) may be of benefit to some. In my experience, this product has not been very effective. Activated charcoal capsules are available over the counter and can be purchased at Walgreens. When activated charcoal is referred to, it does not mean charcoal briquettes used for barbeque grills.

Do not give charcoal barbeque briquettes. Walmart and CVS have the product Charco Caps, but this name is a bit deceiving. This product is not activated charcoal and cannot be expected to do what activated charcoal does. Charco Caps may be effective, but I cannot give you a thumbs-up with this product because I have not tried this product for flatulence prevention. You may choose to give it a try.

The activated charcoal will cause stools to be black. When you see black in the feces, you know your dose is at work. A dose is one to four capsules, depending on the size of the pet. Unfortunately, there is no one dose for each pet; one has to evaluate the effectiveness of the dosage for each pet.

Do not give more than twelve capsules in one day to any dog. Start with the following dosages: small dogs (1–2 capsules), medium dogs (1–7 capsules), and large dogs (1–12 capsules). If you are giving other medications and activated charcoal at the same time, it will reduce the effectiveness of any medication. Therefore, do not give activated charcoal while medicating your pet with any other medications.

PREVENTION

Finding the best diet that produces the least amount gas is the best alternative. Reserve the use of activated charcoal for only when needed.

CONSTIPATION

This is not a common problem for dogs or cats, but it does occur in both. Constipation is an infrequent or difficult defecation with the passage of hard or dry feces. This can occur with any disease or condition that might slow passage of materials in the intestines.

In my experience, the main reason for constipation has been the overfeeding of bones to dogs. In cats, the most common cause is the grooming process creating hairballs. Bone consumption and hair or hairballs are responsible for slowing the movements of the intestinal contents, creating a slow accumulation of intestinal materials within the intestines, resulting in constipation. This is not saying that there are no other causes for the development of constipation.

Signs most often noted with constipation include straining to defecate with small or no fecal volume being expelled. Hard or dry feces, infrequent defecation, small amounts of liquids and/or mucous being discharged, and perhaps small amounts of blood or streaks of blood can be seen.

Besides eating bones and hairballs, it may be due to eating dirt, rocks, feces, or other items. Consumption of excess fiber sources and lack of water have been seen as causes of constipation.

TREATMENT

First, if a dog is being fed lots of bones, stop it completely. The easiest and one of the more effective results is to feed pets undiluted Carnation or Pet condensed/evaporated milk. This normally works within hours as the pet will expel loose feces. Sometimes a Fleet Enema must be completed; with impacted bones, it may take excessive enema treatments to dislodge the dried bones that have impacted the intestines.

PREVENTION

In cats, it is not possible to prevent grooming. A once-in-a-while routine feeding of one of the condensed milk products without dilution will keep the constipation away. Grooming cats is a big help also. In dogs that are fed more than their share of bones, the feeding of bones will need to be stopped. Also if the dog is consuming other objects, those objects need to be eliminated or removed so the dog cannot get to them.

DIFFICULTY SWALLOWING (DYSPHAGIA)

This is not a common issue, but occurs more frequently in dogs than in cats. The leading reason for this problem is an oversized esophagus (megaesophagus). Megaesophagus will normally cause a pet to regurgitate before the food has a chance to get to the stomach. Megaesophagus, or oversized esophagus, is caused by lack of nerves innervating the esophagus. Unfortunately there are no treatments that provide nerve innervation to an enlarged esophagus.

Another issue may be due to a simple blockage within the mouth. There may be pain associated with trying to eat (loose teeth), grabbing the food to allow the pet to chew, or attempting to swallow.

Brain or central nervous system failures may also cause difficulty in swallowing, as well as the inability to grab food. Foreign bodies in the mouth and abnormal developments of the oral cavity may also be reasons for difficulty in swallowing. Congenital malformations include pets with cleft palates. Other medical causes found to be primary causes of difficulty swallowing and regurgitation include esophageal infections and tumors.

Signs that might be observed include drooling, gagging, weight loss, ravenous appetite, repeated attempts to swallow with the head in a normal feeding position, or swallowing with the head in an unusual position.

TREATMENT
If there are foreign bodies in the mouth, they need to be removed. The best treatment for megaesophagus is putting the food higher than usual so the head and neck are in an upward position. The food essentially goes downhill into the stomach.

PREVENTION
Distinguish between vomiting and regurgitation to determine esophageal issues. Vomiting is associated with abdominal contractions, and regurgitation has no abdominal contraction. It is a result of food entering the esophagus and being discharged before reaching the stomach.

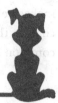

CHAPTER 5

BEHAVIOR

To find fault is easy; to do better may be difficult.
—Plutarch (AD 46–120)

Pet behavior problems are a common owner complaint. Surveys of pet owners reveal that more than 90 percent complain about their dog's behavior. Often, these problems result in pet owners relinquishing their pets to animal shelters.

Behavior of dogs and cats begins at a young age, and it is important that both receive lots of handling and kind treatment. It is beneficial to both cats and dogs if the pet is given the opportunity to develop litter interactions and play as well. Socialization periods for cats are shorter than for dogs. Cat's socialization effectiveness often starts to decline by seven to nine weeks versus a dog, which can range from three weeks to fourteen weeks.

During these short handling and litter interaction periods, dogs and cats may overcome fear and these periods cause both to have less aggressive tendencies. These traits are important as pets become a part of our families. It is also interesting that cats have surpassed dogs as the most popular pet in many countries. Households with children are most likely to have pets, and a majority of pet owners have more than one pet.

The next largest group of pet owners is retired couples. Pets are known to fill many support functions within a household. The behavior of pets becomes all the more important, from feeding, exercising, playing, and being family companions—and perhaps a best buddy. Pets have many health benefits for pet owners, which makes behavior all the more important to pet owners. Within this chapter, the goal is to present some socialization issues as well as other common behaviors.

THE PICKY, PICKY, PICKY EATER

Do you have a picky eater? Many animals can be picky eaters, but the cause of this is taught to the pet by the owner. Here's a common scenario: You feed the foods that you want to feed to your pet. However, you start to feed some treats (Greenies, for example) and maybe some table scraps. When the pet likes the treats and the table food, you continue to feed the purchased food that you want the pet to eat. Alas, you find the pet will not eat the food you want it to eat. Then you cave in and give more special treats or table foods—and the pet eats it all. You have just taught the pet that by waiting a little while, you will feed treats or table food that the pet is waiting on or begging for. This is perhaps the most common cause of the picky eating. Of course, it is not the only cause.

What can you do before jumping off the deep end with this syndrome? One should rule out systemic disease to make sure that you have identified the right syndrome. This is done by testing for pancreatic, dental, gastrointestinal, kidney, or liver disease—all of which can cause picky eating in pets.

Medications may lower food consumption. Blood tests normally need to be completed at your pet's doctor's facility. Once it is known that disease processes are not involved, then the daily food consumption needs to be determined to see if too much food is being fed. Overfeeding can be a cause of not eating.

Many pets will skip a day of eating and still maintain proper weight. Stress in cats can cause anorexia. For example, adding new pets, significant changes in the home, family issues, additions, and schedule changes can be causes. Dental issues are at the top of the list for picky eating. If the pet is an outside pet, make sure it is not getting food from the neighbors. Neighbors feeding animals is a very common occurrence. I have noted this especially with cats. This is due to many people in a neighborhood putting food out for feral cats. If the pet is overweight or holding its correct weight, you may be concerned about what you think is a picky eater—but it is not the issue.

I have noted that lots of pets are given free choice and get way too much food all at once. You need to adjust the amounts you feed so the amounts you feed per day are actually consumed. Do not let foods sit in food dishes for days on end. When I put food down for our cat, the bottom of the dish can always be seen. You should do the same.

Often owners have preconceived ideas of how much should be fed, and it is often an unrealistic expectation. Focus on daily caloric requirements and body weight. Check weight regularly for weight gain or loss. Look in chapter 4 under "Keeping My Pet's Weight Correct." You can keep the correct weight by following those guidelines.

The good news is that most animals will not intentionally starve. However, pets need you to help them be healthy. Instead of feeding cats in a single, regular location, meals may be divided into three or more portions and hidden in various corners, shelves, nooks, and crannies on a rotating basis. In addition, particularly delectable treats may be hidden in different locations on a regular basis. These suggestions can be added to by your own innovations to help the picky eater.

TREATMENT

Pets with medical issues obviously need to have the medical condition treated. Sometimes a switch to a food with less chloric concentration is of benefit as the pet needs to eat more to get to daily caloric needs. Try different things to see if you hit upon one that works for your pet.

1. Moisten dry food with warm water or add some canned food.
2. Adding flavors to the food often helps. Dogs often prefer beef, chicken, lamb, and pork. Choose the one that the pet seems to

like the best. Cats seem to go for chicken, fish, and beef—or perhaps pork. Added gravy seems to be liked a lot; they eat the gravy and leave the foods, particularly cats.

3. Try foods with different flavors. Some do not like to try new things. If the pet will not go for the new food, mix a little of the old with it. Gradually increase the new and decrease the old.

4. Warming the food can bring out aromas and enhance some flavors.

5. Not all animals will respond; some may need the help of the pet's doctor.

6. Treats and other foods can be given in small amounts and must be a small part of the total daily rations to be given.

7. Rather than feed at a single, regular location, meals may be divided into three or more portions and hidden in various corners, shelves, nooks, and crannies on a rotating basis. In addition, particularly delectable treats may be hidden in different locations on a regular basis.

PREVENTION

The one thing you can do is to be aware of the fact that owners often set the stage for nondisease picky eating; understand the causes of nondisease picky or finicky eating of pets.

CATS, CLAWS, AND FURNITURE

Many cats have problems with clawing at furniture, drapes, curtains, and other objects in a house, causing consternation and frustration. Some people will put up with this rather than disposing of the pet. Another issue may be chewing and ingesting things, such as watch batteries, string, needles, and other objects. Our cat likes to take ballpoint pens, pocket knives, and other small objects and hide them under throw rugs. It's amazing what we have found under throw rugs, but it is also very frustrating to come home and find a big hole in a curtain that the cat chewed up or clawed to pieces.

Kittens at five to six weeks of age can wander around the house unsupervised and find all kinds of things to chew on. Some folks think it is funny and provide old chewing shoes, etc. This kind of behavior is often encouraged by the owner. These kinds of events let the cat know it is okay to chew on shoes. Watch out—your best shoes will be next.

Cats like to chew on plants. Make sure you have no poisonous plants around that can kill or make the cat sick. Often plant materials will stimulate vomiting, and you have that to contend with. If extension cords get chewed on, the cat can be burned or killed. You may find other potential things around the house to eliminate or hide from your cat.

TREATMENT

Chewing and scratching behaviors need to be stopped immediately; these items must be put away so the cat cannot get to them. Look around the house for potential chew items and put them away or in areas the cat cannot get to. Keep certain doors closed so the cat cannot get in to destroy the drapes or curtains. This needs to be accomplished for the first year to year and a half.

I do not allow them to be available to young or old cats. Thread kills cats, and needles can get stuck in the throat. Whatever they chew on needs to be eliminated or at least hidden from the cat. Do not encourage young cats to chew on old shoes or other items; it becomes a learned habit that may never be overcome. Supervision is always advised—but is not always able to be provided. Pay attention to the cat by grooming, playing, and spending time with the cat; this seems to help, but it is not a complete solution. This applies to clawing at items as well as chewing or eating drapes and other items.

Some folks swear by a scratching post, but it may be a training post for scratching at other things. Others have no success with scratching posts. This behavior reveals that what works for one will not necessarily work for all cats. If you're a keep-the-claws-on person and can identify the type of materials that the cat seems to attack and scratch at couches, chairs, or curtains, you can get a scratching post.

Take the materials the cat likes to scratch and place them by the area most often attacked or scratched. It is estimated that 20 percent of pet cats are scratchers—and often a solution is never found. In areas where declaws are illegal, the cats often are put into shelters.

PREVENTION

The best prevention is to learn as early as possible if the issues of scratching, chewing, or eating things are noted. Start your program immediately. Do not wait or allow a training period of chewing or scratching. You can also check with your pet's doctor or a veterinarian with special interests in this behavior. He or she might be able to assist. Also an animal trainer who trains cats may be helpful in these situations.

DISTURBING BEHAVIORS FOR DOGS

I have struggled with what to call this discussion since it covers dogs jumping up on people, barking too much, chewing on furniture, destructive chewing, and digging in the yard. This discussion is provided due to the fact that these issues are quite common for pet owners. This discussion is about issues seen more commonly in dogs than in cats.

Most often, these events occur when the pet owner is not home. The owner comes home to a destroyed couch, a dug-up yard, or a hole in the back fence. Your friends come over for a visit, and your dog jumps up on the visitors or barks a lot at them. This can cause embarrassing moments for you and may make your guests wish they had not come over.

Animal behaviorists would lump this issue under canine destructive behavior. They have about the same approach to overcoming these issues. The issues are somewhat complex and need the help of a professional trainer who is familiar with what training is necessary to get the pet to overcome these problems.

The very first is personal commitment and patience, patience, patience. Persistence and consistency are required, and the owner must be willing to work with and spend the time necessary to overcome these types of issues. There is no guarantee that the pet may revert to its habits more than once before the issues are overcome. If the issues are ignored without correctional training, they can become learned behavior. That makes it much harder to train to overcome the unruly behavior.

TREATMENT

If you are good at animal training, you might be able to do it on your own. However, the average pet owner will need to seek professional training help. Petco and PetSmart offer training courses that you can participate in. You should discuss the issues your pet has with the trainer. The trainer may have special sessions with you and your pet. These types of pets have special needs and are not of the general nature of lots of training classes. The trainer needs to focus on your pet's issues and learn all he or she can about your pet's habits and your availability at home to help your pet. It is going to take a team to overcome the pet's challenges. You need to know the capabilities of the trainer before getting started rather than finding out that the trainer is not equipped to handle the type of training you want for your pet.

PREVENTION

There is no specific prevention. However, the sooner you get the training started, the better chance you have of overcoming these types of problems. Do not wait; delaying is bad and reduces the chances of resolving the pet's issues. It is time to get started as soon as you identify the problem; waiting breeds learned behavior, and the behavior becomes introduced in your pet's mind as normal behavior.

WEIRD THINGS DOGS SWALLOW

It is amazing what some dogs manage to swallow. Many are hard to believe that the dog actually swallowed them. I remember reading an article in the 1970s in the *American Veterinary Medical Association Journal (AVMAJ)* with a radiograph of a dog that had swallowed a very large butcher knife that was stuck in the esophagus. The sharp edge of the blade was on top of the dog's heart.

In veterinary college, Dr. Hugh Butler, a surgery professor, showed us photographs of a dog that had swallowed twenty-five feet of half-inch rope. It was all completely wrapped through the dog's intestines.

When I was in Okinawa, an emergency arrived. A lady with a dog said she had just observed the dog swallow twelve feet of cloth. I thought, *Sure, lady, sure.* I gave the dog an emetic—and sure enough the dog vomited up the twelve feet of cloth. The cloth was about five inches wide and twelve feet long. I was dumbfounded, but there it was. She could have induced vomiting at home had she known what and how to do it.

Without supervision and with so many foreign objects accessible to dogs, one cannot judge what a dog might try to eat or swallow. Therefore, it is always best to have the pet under your supervision. When it is impossible to supervise your pet, make sure dangerous objects are put away.

The butcher knife referred to above was deep into the dog's body and could not be reached by hand without anesthesia. Even with anesthesia, it was difficult to retrieve the knife. If it had been simply pulled out, it would have sliced the esophagus and the heart—and there would have been a dead dog. The dog with the twenty-five feet of rope died at home. The dog with the twelve feet of cloth could have been treated at home with little or no problems. The saving grace for the dog with the cloth was that the owner observed the last part of the cloth going into the dog and quickly found veterinary help.

The bottom line is that animals are inquisitive and will explore, chew, and swallow some of the strangest things, which seems impossible. If pets are supervised, swallowing foreign objects does not happen at all. If it is observed, you will know what the issue is—and you might be able to aid your pet immediately. However, if you feel uncomfortable or feel it is beyond your ability, it is best to let your veterinarian handle the issue for you.

TREATMENT

If one knows what was eaten or swallowed—and if the owner knows that introducing vomiting will discharge the item from the stomach *safely*—then vomiting can be induced by giving 3 percent hydrogen peroxide to the dog at a dose of .5 cc to 1 cc of body weight up to a maximum of 2.5 cc per pound of body weight; 3 percent hydrogen peroxide will most often induce vomiting in dogs but not in cats. If hydrogen peroxide is used, you can mix equal parts of milk with the hydrogen peroxide since it helps you to get the hydrogen peroxide down into the stomach.

It is best to discuss what you are about to do with the pet's doctor if possible, or you can call a poison control center. The pet poison helpline free telephone number is 1-800-213-6680. The best solution is to take the pet to see the pet's doctor or to an emergency veterinary facility.

PREVENTION

Make sure the areas in which your dog is allowed to roam do not have items that might be consumed. It could be a life-or-death situation, and your dogs are your buddies. Make sure your pet stays with you for years to come and help your pet be healthy. Certainly direct supervision is the best option for the pet. It protects the pet from trauma and keeps unexpected expenses down.

CAT AND DOG FIGHTS

Unfortunately, cats fight cats, dogs fight dogs, and cats and dogs fight. Most often, both parties receive bites and scratch wounds. These wounds often result in infections on different parts of their bodies.

Large-dog attacks on cats and smaller dogs can cause tremendous damage and often kill cats and smaller dogs. Many wounds caused by larger dogs on smaller cats or dogs are deep and cannot be seen due to the trauma being hidden by the skin. Often there are tear wounds or rip wounds in the abdominal muscles and damage to internal organs. In addition, the muscles over the ribcage can be badly torn—and there can be lung damage. At times, the trauma is adjacent to the diaphragm, allowing organs from the abdomen to become displaced into the thorax with the lungs. Sadly, these kinds of wounds can often be the cause of death for cats and smaller dogs.

Cat fights between cats most often result in abscesses on different parts of the body. The most frequent areas of abscesses are found in areas that are bitten or scratched. Obviously a bite or scratch can be anywhere on the pet's body. Cat fight wounds tend to be on the front of the front legs, top of the head, and the ears. The belly and just forward of the tail may also be targets in a cat fight. Experience with cat fights shows the most frequent area of fight abscesses to be just anterior to the tail head, in the region of the tail head, or in or around the tail head. The tail head is where the tail is attached to the body. Often the signs noted are draining from a bite that has become infected and popped open because the infectious materials (exudates) are being discharged.

Dog fights between dogs, depending on the size of the dogs involved, normally determine the varying degrees of severity inflicted due to the bites and/or scratches. Dog fight wounds left untreated—just like cat bites—will become infected and may cause very large areas of swelling due to infection of connective and cellular tissues (cellulitis).

The pain from bites can be so severe that the pet will be lame in a leg if it becomes infected. Medical treatment after a confrontation can prevent infection and tissue swelling. The most common areas of trauma after a dog fight are on the face, head, neck, and anterior of the front legs. If a dog turns to run, it may be bitten on the rear legs or back. However, rear bites on dogs seem to be rare. The ears can be badly damaged and bleed a lot. If you happen to have QuikClot or PetClot available, you can stop bleeding fast. Dogs and cats often bite or scratch wounds of people; this is discussed later in this book.

TREATMENT

The best treatment plan is to take your pet to see the pet's doctor; medication should be given to prevent infections from occurring. It is much easier and much cheaper to treat right after a confrontation than to wait and have to treat abscesses. It is also much better for the pet's health. It will save you money due to the extra medications, such as fluids and others that may be needed if you wait to have your pet treated.

PREVENTION

The best prevention is to always have your pet on a leash when outside. The problem I have noted is when another dog is not on a leash and the dog attacks your dog.

BITTEN BY YOUR PET

It may come as a surprise that owners are frequently bitten by their pets—sometimes rather severely. We will discuss some of the frequencies and results of pets biting their owners—but not the psychology about why they bite.

Of all bites, 51 percent are from cats, 40 percent of bites are from dogs, and the rest are from other animals. Pet bites are most often unprovoked. For example, I know a person who was reading in bed with her cat. She looked down, and her cat jumped at her face and bit her next to the left eye. No reason could be determined about why the cat attacked, and the bite was close to inflicting damage to the owner's eye. At a later date, the cat attempted to bite her face again, but she had her book and defended herself. Unfortunately, the cat had to be disposed of.

At our facility, many dogs are turned in due to bites. The facility only has fifteen bite runs for dogs that have bitten people—either owned or nonowned. These runs are always full, and each dog has a history of attacking and/or biting. Sadly, some people are badly bitten. The largest percentages of dog bites, about 90 percent, are due to pit bulls.

When I was doing a tour of duty at the Military Dog Center at Lackland Air Force Base, we would often go to Europe to purchase military working dogs. The Belgian police were using Rottweilers as police dogs. A policeman dog handler was on duty at a lookout and happened to drop a sandwich between the dog's front legs. The policeman bent over to retrieve the sandwich, and the dog attacked him. He had to shoot the dog to get it off.

Another incident occurred with a Doberman pinscher at Lackland Air Force Base. An air policeman had been handling his dog for quite some time. One evening, he bent over to pet the dog, which was a normal part of their relationship. For some reason, the dog jumped at the handler and bit his nose off. Doctors at Wilford Hall Hospital at Lackland Air Force Base were able to sew the nose back on. However, the dog could no longer be trusted with any handler.

We get animals in for surgery because the owners are afraid of the pet and are completely unable to control it. This pet may cause a large number of bites to animal owners and non–animal owners. Furthermore, they are often the types of dogs who attack other dogs in neighborhoods.

TREATMENT

In most cases of animals with biting and attacking issues, retraining is beyond the ability of most owners, and professional help is needed. You may get help from your veterinary behaviorist or with a professional animal trainer.

Some pets are only good with the owner and no one else. If someone attempts to do anything with the pet, they are either bitten or mauled. Be aware of such animals—and do not attempt to pet or befriend this type of animal. I know a person who attempted such a thing and lost an arm and was almost killed by the dog. A strong suggestion is to stay away and leave strange, snarling dogs alone. The pet that never bites anyone is a perfect candidate for biting. I have been bitten by dogs that supposedly had never bitten anyone. Be wise—not painful and bleeding. Keeping your hands to yourself and away from strange dogs will prevent biting incidents.

Some cats have what is known as "petting-induced aggression." After petting a cat with this habit for a period of time, the cat decides it has had enough petting and will bite. Sometimes the bite is hard and may cause bleeding. Just pet the cat for a short time—and then leave it alone.

Sometimes a cat may bite when you stop petting. Anticipate this behavior and take a break from the animal. Maybe that is a good time to go get a drink of water or make some popcorn; when you come back, most often the cat will have moved. This trick seems to work quite well.

PREVENTION

Some animals have food aggression or aggression toward other animals. You need to be aware of this; do not allow the opportunity for these types of behavior to occur. You can do this by avoiding the pet's food while the pet is eating. You also need to let others know that the pet has this problem. If a pet sitter comes over and is mauled, it is not a pleasant experience for the owner or the pet sitter. It would be a terrible experience for a pet sitter to be bitten or mauled simply because you did not tell the sitter your pet is food aggressive and to leave the pet's food alone if the pet is eating.

If a pet has food aggression, when a person attempts to move a food bowl, that person will probably be bitten or mauled. As for other animal aggression, do not allow others to come close or allow the pet to be off of a leash in the outside. An animal-aggressive dog allowed to run loose is foreboding and is a problem just waiting to happen.

Cats attempt the same things, but are not large enough to maul. Keep in mind that their bites and scratches can be very painful. I know of a case that resulted in both legs being amputated due to an infected cat bite on an arm. *How the heck could the legs be involved from a bite on the arm?* I cannot answer that, but I know it happened. With any animal bite, you need to see your physician because bites by dogs and cats have caused many people to be hospitalized for treatment. It can be a very serious situation. As reminder, unprovoked biting by animals could be due to rabies.

SKUNKS AND PETS

The funny thing about skunks is that they seem not to have any natural enemies; even poisonous snakes know better than to mess with skunks. It is believed this lack of fear in skunks is why they get themselves into places where they may be run over or hurt badly.

I have been sprayed by skunks in cold weather and did not realize I had been sprayed until I walked into the warm house—and then it smelled like the skunk was in the house. The smell is pungent. I have been asked about skunks spraying pets by Canadians, and I add this short blurb for the friends up north. I assume that there are more skunk issues in Canada than in the United States. Before starting the termination of skunk odor, check the pet's eyes to see if they are red; if so, the pet may have been sprayed in the eyes. The spray will not hurt the eyes, but it is definitely not comfortable for the pet. You may need a bit of help from your pet's doctor. Washing the eyes with water would benefit the pet—just as it is for a pet that has been sprayed in the eyes by a cobra.

If you do not have the following on hand, you will need to run to the grocery store or pharmacy to obtain the items necessary to mix together a remedy for your pet. I call this remedy the "terminator" of skunk odor. Get one tube of artificial tears ointment to put into the eyes just before pouring or sponging your terminator on your pet's head. You will need a clean bucket or large pan to mix the solution: one quart of hydrogen peroxide (if it is a big dog, perhaps two or three quarts), baking soda, and dishwashing or laundry soap of some kind. Because this mixture is so reactive, for safety reasons do not mix it in a bottle. *Do not save any leftovers.*

When the solution is mixed and you are about to treat your pet, there are a few things you need to take care of first. First, put an artificial tears ointment in the pet's eyes as a partial protection from getting any of the solution in the eyes. Wet the pet down with warm water if possible. Put on disposable rubber gloves and pour your terminator solution on your pet. When you do the pet's head, hold your hand over the eyes so you can prevent as much of the solution as possible from getting into the eyes or use a sponge to do the head of your pet.

Follow these steps:

- The mixture will need to be mixed in a clean bucket or a large bowl. Do not mix in a bottle or small container because the ingredients are very reactive. Use disposable rubber gloves to apply the terminator mixture.
- Add one quart of hydrogen peroxide to one quart of water.
- Add .25 (1/4) cup of Arm and Hammer baking soda (sodium bicarbonate).

- Add 1–2 teaspoons of any liquid soap (dish or laundry soap will do well).
- Mix solution with a plastic utensil.
- Use disposable rubber gloves to protect your hands.
- Wet the pet just before applying the terminator (with warm water if possible).
- Pour the terminator mixture on the pet and work it into the hair down to the skin.
- When you are ready to poor the solution on the head, hold your hand over the eyes to help protect them. It may be desirable to use a sponge on the head and face, being careful to prevent the solution from getting into the eyes of your pet. You may not be able to remove the entire odor from the face, but do your best with what you have.
- Let the terminator mixture sit on the animal for about ten minutes.
- Keep your pet from licking at the solution and rinse off after ten minutes.
- Discard any excess solution. Do not save since it is very reactive.

CATS SPRAYING URINE

Spraying urine is a method of marking territory by female and male cats. Male cats tend to express this behavior more often than female cats. The event usually occurs when the cat begins smelling something (a wall, furniture, or rug) and turns and sprays in that area. This is the most common misbehavior of cats. Urinating outside the litter box is a behavior normally found when the litter box is dirty and needs to be cleaned. A dirty litter box may lead to permanently urinating outside the litter box. Another stimulus for urinating out of the litter box is a urinary tract infection. Even though dirty litter boxes and urinary tract infections are frequent occasions for urinating out of the litter box, this discussion will focus on spraying or marking territory with urine. When marking territory, cats stand to void a small amount of urine for the purpose of marking and establishing their territory. This behavior is also a method of leaving their claim on the territory to let other cats that approach the territory know that a urine-marked claim has been established. This behavior can be annoying to owners and frequently leads to disposing of the cat or having to put it to sleep.

Cats tend to like areas with lower populations of cats, and each will tend to mark territory. Spraying is most frequently done on vertical or horizontal surfaces. Often the cat will back up to the spot to urinate while holding their tail in a vertical, quivering position. These behavior patterns are often used as key signs that the spraying is for the purpose of marking territory. Households with more than one cat are left to determine which cat or cats are the culprit in the spraying syndrome.

TREATMENT

Neutering male and female cats seems to be the best alternative for spraying cats. Male neutering will normally be successful for 80 percent of male cats. Another 10 percent of the male cats will stop spraying about two or three months after being neutered. Spaying of females can be effective too, but it is not as well documented. These figures will differ according to different authors and experiences of different practices—and they are not necessarily the alpha and omega of cat urine spraying data.

PREVENTION

There have been many ideas presented about what stimulates a cat to start spraying, and the list seems to grow. Causes of this behavior include new cats in the area of an established household cat, dirty litter boxes, avoiding litter boxes that creates punishment (such as very small litter pans, little or no litter in the pan, never cleaning the pan), large numbers of cats in a household (ten or more), houses with only male cats, and stress. Trying to avoid these stimuli should be the goal of a person presented with this issue.

BITING BODY PARTS

This is a syndrome of unknown cause that occurs occasionally and almost exclusively in dogs. It is very rare in cats. It is unknown about why dogs bite, chew, and eat different body parts, such as the tail, leg, foot, or penis, but the bottom line is that no one seems to know why dogs are constantly biting at themselves. It is obvious when watching a dog bite at itself that the bite is painful, but why the dog keeps biting at itself is unknown. For owners that have this problem in a pet, it is frustrating and terrifying condition for which there is currently no known cure.

Suggestions for the stimulus for the start of the biting mutilation syndrome are numerous, and many theories are listed as possible causes. None seem to be a real initiating factor and are presented as ideas that might be causes, which adds to the frustration concerning the condition.

TREATMENT

Amputation has been tried on certain parts of the body. However, when the part being bitten is removed, the biting restarts higher up. Therefore, the removal of a body part seems to have no effect on the biting and chewing on body parts. There currently is no effective treatment for biting mutilation. For a palliative treatment, an Elizabethan collar can be placed to prevent the dog from getting to part of the body, and bandages can be applied to the wounds. This is probably a lifetime sentence with an Elizabethan collar, however.

PREVENTION

As the cause of the self-biting syndrome is unknown, there is nothing that can be done to prevent the biting syndrome from occurring. Maybe the good news is that this syndrome is not common. Ouch!

GETTING A LOST PET BACK HOME

Many pets are allowed outside without supervision. This allows a pet to wander off into strange territory and not be able to find their way home. It is surmised that folks believe that all pets are Lassie-Come-Home types, but they could not be more wrong. Just this week, a lady informed me that she opened the door—and her cat slipped out into the abyss of the outdoors. Two days later, the cat has not returned.

How do you find your pet?

Another cat got out and climbed onto an engine of a car that was driven seventeen miles before the driver stopped to look at what was making the noise under the hood. The poor cat was fried and in severe pain. The reality is that neither owner will ever get their pets back.

What do people do? They resort to a photo on a bulletin board. Just how many bulletin boards are there in any community that people actually look at? Unfortunately, even with one hundred bulletin boards, the chances of finding a pet this way are like winning the Powerball lottery. It just does not happen other than by accident. There are much better ways of finding a pet. I've listed them from poor to the best:

- The worst identification on any pet is absolutely nothing.
- Rabies tags are not quite as bad as having no identification, but they are in the same ballpark.
- How many pets have rabies tags? Where did they get it—and when?
- Identification tags with telephone numbers and addresses are great if the collar holding the tags has not fallen off or been removed. What if it was not on the pet when it disappeared?
- Unregistered identification chips can be placed under the skin. Sometimes the source of the chip can be found, and a pet can be identified by the installing organization.
- A registered identification chip placed under the skin works well.

TREATMENT

The best way to get your pet back is if you have an identification chip put under the skin of your pet. You can call and register the number of the chip. The telephone number for the National Pet Microchip

Registration (RFID-USA™) is 1-866-211-9590. The fax number is 1-800-278-2114, and the website is http://registermicrochip.com.

PREVENTION

There are literally thousands of pets that have wandered off or gotten out of homes that become lost and are never found. Some are run over, killed, starved, or dehydrated; others get skin diseases, end up in shelters, or maybe find new homes. Those that find a new home might be one in twenty. Do not let your pet be one of these—and take action before it is too late.

BITING ELECTRIC CORDS

The idea that a pet would bite on an electric cord may seem unthinkable, but it does happen every once in a while. You do not want to be the owner of a pet that has the misfortune of biting into a charged electric wire. The most common pet to do this is a young dog (aged five to eighteen months). That does not rule out younger or older ages from similar occurrences.

The young are investigating lots of things, and an electric wire out in the area is a fun item to chew on. This is a very rare event in cats. One would think that playful cats would be more likely to bite on wires. Regardless of the animal, it is a good idea to not have electric wires exposed in areas that are open to pets. The other option is to not allow young pets into areas that have exposed electric wires, including holiday electric cords. The good news is that there are very few other opportunities for pets to be accidentally electrocuted.

Injury due to electric cord biting can be rather severe for the pet. Perhaps the most common injury due to chewing on electric cords is burns in the mouth and lips. There is always a chance that the electric charge may affect the heart. Though an uncommon occurrence, it can cause heart failure due to the jolt of the electric charge. The electric charge can cause fluids to accumulate in the lungs, and there have been cases involving pulmonary hypertension, which is an increase in the pet's blood pressure in the lungs. Some pets have developed cataracts due to an electric charge from chewing on electric cords.

Signs you might observe in a dog that has received an electric shock include burns of the gums or cheek tissues, singed hair and whiskers, and difficulty breathing. Perhaps the most common sign noted is coughing and an increased rate of breathing. In some cases of electrocution, the gums or mucous membranes of the mouth may be pale or bluish, which may include muscle tremors or collapsing.

TREATMENT

As you have learned above, there can be a range of issues involved in biting extension cords or other electric cords. The treatment requirement may be for a simple burn on the lips, or there may be major health issues due to fluids in the lungs or heart problems. If the electric shock is minor, such as singed hair and whiskers, there is not much to do. On the other hand, there may be a need for a visit to the pet's doctor to make sure all is well. If necessary, take other appropriate steps to treat the pet.

PREVENTION

The ideal prevention is to eliminate any possibility of the young pet finding wires to chew on by keeping wires out of areas that the pets are allowed into or preventing the pet from entering areas that have electric wires.

CHAPTER 6

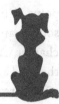

BRAINS AND NERVES

We need men who can dream of things that never were.
—John F. Kennedy

There are many, many different types and causes of brain or peripheral nerve issues. There are so many that they are too numerous to list. All kinds of things can go wrong with brains and nerves. Those parts that include the brain and the spinal cord are commonly referred to as the central nervous system (CNS).

The many nerves that go to different parts of the body all have names. Every part of a body has a nerve stimulus of some kind. The nerves to different parts of the body may allow feeling or allow movement. Other nerves can have both components in the same nerve.

I guess one could look upon the nervous system as a road map. The CNS might be considered to be a large metropolitan area, and the nerves outside the metropolitan area are the highways. As you know, traffic accidents can occur in metropolitan areas as well on highways—and the same is true with the nervous system. Accidents can occur in the CNS or the nerve network.

When there is a traffic accident in the metropolitan area or on a highway (or in this case, nerves or CNS), traffic stops. It is the same in the nerve network. There will be no feeling or ability to move due to blockage of traffic or nerve impulses. The pet will show signs of nerve damage, which might be lameness or the inability to walk or get up, or seizures. Sometimes a traffic accident allows some traffic to pass the accident but will not allow all traffic to pass. It is the same with nerve damage. Feeling or movement might pass the trauma point. When a pain producer is applied to the pet, the pet may make sounds and not move—or it may move and not have feeling. This chapter will cover a few of the more common problems seen within the road area (nerves) network or problems within the metropolitan (CNS) areas.

PAIN RECOGNITION

Pain in pets is a sign that there is something amiss with the pet, and it should be investigated for the purpose of determining the origin of the pain. The origin may be a simple matter to overcome. On the other hand, it may be a serious issue that requires extensive work to determine the cause of the pain. It must be remembered that cats may have pain but conceal it from view, and they are more apt to do this than dogs are.

Pain reactions by dogs or cats are often based on the personality of the pet and the severity of the pain. Posture may be a sign of pain and may be expressed by a hunched back with a lowered head. The animal may be guarding a painful area of the body part that is causing pain. When the area of pain is touched, the dog may attempt to bite. A dog may put its front end down with the head between the front legs and keep the rear end up high, attempting to shift its body weight to help limit pain. Also dogs and cats may lie in abnormal positions.

Movements of a pet may cause you to recognize certain signs. Signs noticed might be stiffness, not putting weight on a particular leg or foot, holding up a foot or leg, restlessness, trembling, or shaking. They may have very limited movement while awake.

Some pets will vocalize, and others will be quiet; this is not a routinely noticeable sign in dogs or cats. If the pet is vocal, it will normally be loud and easily recognized as pain. Cats may hiss, growl, or bite if painful areas of the body are examined by palpation or touching. Some dogs are quick to bite if painful areas are palpated or touched; caution is essential when dealing with pets in pain. Some dogs will let you touch, move, and palpate until the cows come home.

Personalities are different. There may also be nerve damage associated with the trauma.

Behavioral changes may be noted or present. Do not hang your hat on behavioral changes, but if they are present, they may not be apparent. Some behavioral changes include agitated attitude, limited or poor grooming, poor appetite or lack of drinking water, acting out of character, licking at wounds (which normally makes the wound worse), and hiding.

Pain may be caused by being hit by a car, bites, or other such traumas. There are chronic low-grade pains due to disease or systemic body malfunctions, such as kidney failure, pancreatitis, fatty liver syndrome, and others.

TREATMENT

Most frequently, the pain-producing issues are not treatable by owners. There may be broken bones, deep infections, or infected skin wounds. As for systemic issues, they have to be diagnosed by test and often require special tests to determine the cause of the pain. Minor skin wounds can be treated with a triple antibiotic ointment, and there are several brands available at grocery stores, CVS, Walgreens, and Walmart.

PREVENTION

Prevention of a specific trauma or systemic cause is hard due to the fact that it is not possible to predict the future of any living organism. Systemic body malfunctions, such as diabetes, pancreatic inflammation (pancreatitis), cancers, and others make a good preventive medicine program a great idea. A good preventive medicine pet program can catch these kinds of issues early and save you big bucks. When dealing with animals in pain, they will bite to let you know it is hurting. Be careful when dealing with pets in pain. They will bite an owner just as fast as a nonowner.

SMALL DEVELOPED CEREBELLUM OF THE BRAIN (CEREBELLA HYPOPLASIA)

This is a syndrome that occurs in the uterus before birth. The cerebellum of the brain does not develop normally due to the disease panleukopenia virus (feline distemper) exposure occurring in the uterus about the time of birth or shortly before birth. Signs become evident as soon as the animal is able to walk. This includes a wide stance, whole body tremors, unsure footing (ataxia), and stumbling. Depending on the severity of the nonprogressive condition, the cat can have a good quality of life if steps are taken to prevent falling—and the cat is kept indoors.

TREATMENT

There is no treatment for the condition once the cat has a small cerebellum. The treatment for this syndrome is preventive. All that is necessary is to immunize cats when they reach the appropriate age for the panleukopenia (feline distemper) immunizations.

PREVENTION

This syndrome is best prevented by vaccinating the cat before pregnancy for panleukopenia virus.

EPILEPSY

Epilepsy is a complex disease, and this discussion is to provide information as a short overview for those pet owners who have pets with this condition. Epilepsy is a brain disorder, which has recurrent seizures in the absence of any abnormal neurological form or structure within the central nervous system or not having any underlying disease process.

This phenomenon is very rare in cats, but it is genetic in many breeds of dogs. Some of the breeds that may be more prone to this type of epilepsy seizure include shepherds, beagles, cocker spaniels, collies and border collies, dachshunds, golden retrievers, Irish setters, and Saint Bernards. Even though there are those that seem to be more prone to seizure activity, it does not exclude any particular breed.

Seizures may be generalized from onset, and there may be some signs that a seizure is about to occur. The preseizure signs are most often referred to as a short aura. The preseizure (or aura) seems to be a frequent sign noted as an onset by many owners of seizing pets. Seizures are considered to be of three basic types—generalized seizures, partial seizures, and partial seizures that turn into generalized seizures. Seizures can be classified as true idiopathic and inherited or as acquired and noninherited. Noninherited epilepsy is normally the result of some type of trauma to the head that produces no neurologic defects other than seizures. Treatment for inherited and noninherited is the same, but long-term results may be better for treated cases of noninherited epilepsy.

Seizures can occur any time, but they often occur while a pet is resting or asleep—and at night or early in the morning. Signs of seizure may include falling to one side, becoming stiff, chomping its jaws, salivating profusely, urinating, defecating, vocalizing, or paddling its legs and feet.

In young dogs, first seizures can occur between six months and five years. The most severe cases of epilepsy normally have an onset of less than two years of age. After a seizure, a pet may have confusion and disorientation, pacing, and other signs. It may take up to twenty-four hours to recover.

Other metabolic conditions may cause seizures, and it is important that a diagnosis be made to ensure that the pet is not epileptic. Blood tests are essential for ruling out other causes.

TREATMENT
This condition requires the diagnostic ability and help of the pet's doctor. This is important for a proper diagnosis and dispensing of the correct medications. Weight gain is often an issue for dogs on epilepsy treatment. If you notice your pet gaining weight, consult your pet's doctor for actions to be taken.

PREVENTION

Epilepsy is an inherited disease, and it is best not to allow breeding of dogs that have epilepsy.

LAMENESS

There are so many causes of lameness that it is difficult to know where to start. The problem with most lameness is that the cause may be difficult to determine—and often needs the aid of the pet's doctor to make the determination. The causes of lameness go on forever. A few things that will cause lameness are a ruptured anterior cruciate, arthritis, old age, hip dysplasia, elbow dysplasia, a luxating patella, broken bones, injured toes, muscle pain, injured toenails, and joint luxation. Also wound infections—such as bite wounds, cuts, grass awns, wound infections of the legs, and many more pain-producing events—can result in painful lameness.

Many lameness cases are not painful. Examples might include old bone fractures that heal improperly. Improper healing of bone fractures can make joints stiff or nonmovable, make one leg shorter than another, or result in missing parts of legs or feet.

Lameness can occur in any age or sex of any animal. The most frequent cause of lameness is trauma of some sort that results in pain to the animal. Trauma cases include being hit by a car, kicked, hit with objects, falling, or being thrown.

Sometimes infections or open wounds are easily noticeable, but others become a question of what the heck is happening. Normally with lameness comes pain. When identifying a lame pet, be aware that the pet may bite if you touch a painful spot.

When examining a pet for lameness, you will find that it is easier to determine lameness in dogs than in cats. Cats tend to sit or stand and look around before moving. In cats, if you suspect a front or rear leg injury, the best thing to do is to hold the cat up and then place the cat on the floor front feet first. If there is pain in one leg, they will normally put the good leg and good foot down first and tend to hold the lame leg up. This can be repeated to examine the rear legs.

In most cases of dog lameness, one can put a leash on the dog and let the dog walk. It will limp on the lame leg or hold a leg up, allowing easy recognition of the leg in question. Often broken bones can be felt in a lame leg. Broken bones hurt; if approached with guerrilla tactics, you will normally be bitten. Be slow, cautious, and easy; bone crepitation can be felt with very little movement.

If at all possible, muzzle a pet you suspect has pain from trauma. Muzzling will save you from unexpected and unwanted bites. Radiology can prove or disprove your observations if one is inclined to obtain confirmation of the cause of leg lameness.

TREATMENT

Treatment depends on the type of trauma that has occurred. Broken bones, gunshot wounds, muscle pain, or infections are examples of pain-producing lameness. One needs to remember that old healed wounds or congenital issues do not necessarily produce pain; they are anatomical or body malformations causing lameness.

If it is a superficial skin wound, triple antibiotic ointment can be applied and bandaged. Triple antibiotic ointments can be purchased at grocery stores, pharmacies, and Walmart. Apply the ointment and bandages until the wound is healed. If it is a deep infection causing large swelling of tissues or draining tracts, broken bones, or other causes, it is a job for the pet's doctor. If it happens to be an old fracture that has healed, perhaps it can be rebroken and treated properly. This type of treatment may be an option. Each improperly healed bone fracture is different and requires different approaches for treatment. It often requires leaving an old fracture the way it is. There is very little that can be done for missing legs, feet, or other body parts. There are some prosthetics that are being produced for pets. New modern pet prosthetics may be an option.

PREVENTION

Since no one knows what the future holds for trauma or lameness, it is impossible to have a program of prevention. However, if you are letting your pet outside without supervision, you can start going with your pet and prevent dog fights, being hit by cars, and other issues. Pet supervision is a good idea always. It saves trauma to pets—and saves money for owners.

INTERVERTEBRAL DISC DISEASE

Unfortunately, intervertebral disc disease is a rather common disease. It is most often seen in dogs, but it does occur in cats. The back bones have a hollow tube (spinal canal) that runs from the brain to the pelvis. In this canal, nerves provide nerve innervations for movement or feeling to different parts of the body. Below the canal or tube that runs within the bones (vertebra) of the back are cushions between each bone of the back.

The cushions provide a space-filling function as well as absorbing jars and jerks in the back. These cushions can be traumatized, affected by age, or damaged. Age and trauma can allow disc eruptions to occur. A very common cause of back disc problems occurs when a pet is hit by a car. Discs that are associated with arthritis or disc degeneration due to age may erupt and move into the spinal nerve canal between the back bones (vertebrae). This can cause pressure on the nerves that are in the back bone canal, which damages nerves in the canal and produces signs of lameness in a pet.

Signs that are noticeable are due to lack of nerve innervation. The most common signs include the inability to use the rear legs, no feelings in the rear legs, or an inability to control urination or defecation. One can pinch the toes; if there is no reaction or movement, this is a bad sign that indicates the pet needs to get to the doctor quickly. These signs occur when a disc ruptures and moves up between bones (vertebrae) in the lower back or so-called lumbar region of the back. Discs can also move up the spinal canal in the neck or in the chest part of the back. Other signs that might be seen include paralysis, inability to walk normally, walking with great difficulty, spinal pain, urinary and fecal incontinence, and loss of feeling.

Signs of an intervertebral disc problem in the neck include neck pain from moving the head back and forth, front limb lameness, or the inability to use the front legs. If the disc problem is in the thorax area, the pet may not be able to use its legs.

Several dog breeds seem to be more prone to this type of spontaneous disease, such as dachshunds (very common), beagles, poodles, cocker spaniels, and Doberman pinschers. This disease can also occur in any breed that receives severe trauma. The most important thing to know about this disease is that it is an emergency. Actions need to happen fast—or the dog will be paralyzed or crippled forever.

This disease needs professional diagnosis and treatment. Delays are catastrophic for a pet. When moving the pet to the pet's doctor's office, handle the pet cautiously—without further traumatizing the back. Do not throw the pet in the car and go. If there is something solid to place the pet on for transport, that is the ideal method of transport for any back or neck injury. Of course, that is not always possible.

TREATMENT

This is an issue for the pet's doctor if the pet is to get well after suffering from disc problems. It is impossible to aid a pet with over-the-counter medications. It is an extreme emergency that needs to be seen by a veterinarian quickly.

PREVENTION

There is little one can do to prevent disc disease. However, if you have a wellness plan with your pet's doctor and if you and the veterinarian think it would be beneficial to take radiographs of the back and neck, this may give clues to potential problems in the future. It can be repeated if necessary for any developing issues. Of course, this is not a normal part of a wellness plan, but if one has a breed that is prone to this disease, it may pay big dividends in the future.

WORMS IN PEOPLE

There was a program on TV in which a physician operated on a woman and removed a worm from her brain. It was due to modern technology that a diagnosis was able to be made by CAT scan or MRI. The bad news is that the worm can also migrate to an eye and cause blindness. The purpose of this article is to describe how such infections occur in people.

The most common sources of these parasites are raccoons and skunks that visit local neighborhoods and public parks at night foraging for food and other things. They bring fleas into yards, and animals might deposit feces in yards or public parks. When deposited, the feces normally contain thousands of parasitic eggs. For raccoons, it is most likely *Baylisascaris procyonis;* for skunks and badgers, it is *Baylisascaris columnaris.* The eggs are very hardy and can last years in different environments. The eggs of these parasites are not hurt by freezing or hot weather changes throughout the year.

In another case, a woman took her child to a public park. The child happened to pick up some feces from a raccoon. The mother saw this happen and removed all that she could. She had the presence of mind to have the sample examined by her physician and Baylisascaris eggs were found. Young children are often infected due to sticking dirt or other objects in their mouths or sticking dirty hands in their mouths. It has been determined that washing hands helps prevent these diseases.

Dogs can also become infected but normally have the parasite in its intestines (as so-called definitive host infection). Some species of dogs, although rare, may have a migrating infection (or so-called paratenic host infection). In dogs, normal roundworm treatments will treat this parasite if it is in the intestinal tract. It is believed that human infestation from dogs has a very low rate of occurrence and may not be of concern. Certainly if the owner has a preventive medicine program, parasites will not normally be of any concern. A second issue with dogs that might have the parasite infection of Baylisascaris in their intestinal tract is the possibility of contaminating the environment when it leaves stools. If the dog gets feces on its hair, it can be a source of infections for family members. Rats can have intestinal Baylisascaris, and if they get into a home, they can leave feces on floors and allow for potential human exposure.

If a dog gets feces on its coat, the feces should be washed off as soon as possible. The problem is you will not know the source of the feces that has gotten onto the dog. If you do not properly wash the dog, you might become infected too. Rubber gloves and a plastic apron are in order to prevent you from getting the disease.

TREATMENT

As for human exposure, diagnosis and treatment is a job for your physician. For animals, all normal roundworm treatments will treat intestinal roundworm infestations. Nonintestinal infections are rare. There is no treatment for the migrating phase of this parasite.

PREVENTION

The best prevention is to be aware. Do not allow young children or pets to roam without proper supervision. Lack of supervision is almost always the cause of trauma and these infestations.

CHAPTER 7

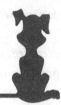

PETS AND POISONS (TOXINS)

*Personally I'm always ready to learn, although
I do not always like being taught.*
—Sir Winston Churchill

Poisons consumed by pets are almost always unknown. Unfortunately, everyone has to start at ground zero about what toxic compound is causing the signs observed in the pet. All anyone knows is that the pet is not doing well. Therefore, if an owner observes consumption or believes he or she knows what the pet has eaten or gotten into, it is important that that information is shared with the poison center or the veterinarian.

Cats are worse than dogs when poisoned because they tend to hide and may not be found until it is too late. A response to a poison depends on several factors that enhance or detract from the poison's ability to cause disease or physical harm. These include the current health of the pet and the amount of the poison consumed or sprayed on the skin. The frequency of consuming the poison, route of exposure, amount consumed, concentration of the poison, how fast it is absorbed into the body, and the ability of the pet to metabolize the poison are important factors.

If a poison was consumed on an empty stomach, absorption will be much quicker than if it had occurred on a full stomach. Very small amounts normally do not present problems. It depends on the type and concentration of the poison. Do not take a chance; for large or small amounts, it is best to get help quickly. Following ingestion or skin contamination, pets will often show early signs by vomiting—particularly if the stomach happens to be empty.

The environment may affect the poison consumed. Barometric pressure, humidity, and temperature affect toxicity of pets due to mycotoxins and excess nitrates in plants due to rain. In this chapter, we will present some subjects on a few common poisons (toxins) that create issues for household pets.

COMMON TOXINS IN THE HOUSE

There are numerous toxic compounds in and around a house. There are so many toxic compounds that there are folks that deal with nothing but toxins. An issue for pet owners is just knowing what the pet happened to eat or get on its body that caused signs of toxicity or death.

Unfortunately, most of the toxic events will occur without your knowledge; often when you see the pet, it is showing signs already or near death. Your veterinarian is a front-line aid for diagnosing and treating your pet. Many toxic compounds can cause similar signs, making a correct identification of the cause difficult.

Your pet's doctor has had rather extensive training in diagnosing the cause by the signs seen in pets. Table 7.1 describes many common toxins found around the house and identifies the compound, organs affected, and toxic elements in the compound that cause the toxicity and describes low-dose and high-dose signs in pets.

I have selected a few toxins that your pet *might* be exposed to. Believe it or not, chocolate is one of the more common toxins for pets. Leaving a box of chocolates out without a weighted lid has resulted in many a pet becoming sick or dying. Pets are expert at opening boxes to get to chocolate, and they tend to consume most of the box. Pets seem to like chocolates a lot and eat them quickly. The toxic compound in the chocolate is theobromine, and smaller amounts of caffeine are methylxanthines. Caffeine is found in coffee, tea, and some diet pills. Signs can occur within an hour of consumption of chocolate. Usually the first signs are vomiting and diarrhea followed by hyper-excitability, weakness, ataxia, seizure, and coma. If that is not enough, it is followed by heart problems, such as premature ventricular contractions and other heart problems, and is followed by death.

The list of toxic compounds and plants is almost limitless and is not the subject of this book. Your pet's doctor is the first line of defense for diagnosis and treatment. In addition, you may contact a poison control center. Almost every state has a poison control center. You can search for "state poison control centers" and find American, Canadian, and Mexican poison control centers rather easily and quickly. The following poison control centers are provided as a reference for you if you need to obtain information on eliminating poisons you think might be in or around your home, or for any other concern you may have about poisons.

The "Pet Poison Helpline" is 1-800-426-4435; the telephone call is free, but they charge a fee of about $35 for consultations. Their free download for smartphones is the best I have seen. It is very easy to use without any instructions and allows the poison you want to look up to be found easily and quickly. In the same field you are looking at to see the effects of the poison, there is a button on the lower right corner to push to call the poison center directly under the subject compound you are looking at. The program is awesome. I like the free download a lot because it is so simple to use.

On your cell phone, go to the App Store. In the app, touch search, and type "Pet Poison Help." The app will come up for free download. The other center is the SPCA 1-888-426-4435; the call is free, and the change for consultation is about $65.

Table 7.1 *Toxic Items around the House*

May Cause Toxicity	Organs Affected	Toxic Compound (Poison)	Mild-Dose Effects	Large-Dose Effects
Sugarless candies, toothpaste, sugar-free gum	Liver damage	Xylitol	Increased insulin production, lower blood sugar levels	Liver failure, bleeding issues— outcome may be death
Grapes and raisins	GI tract, with vomiting and diarrhea	Not identified at this time	Often no signs from 2–4 grapes or raisins— vomiting, diarrhea, lethargy, and refusal to eat	Kidney failure in 24 hours with only 0.32 oz. and 0.50 oz. of raisins. Some eat more with no effects.
Onions (dried or wet) and garlic	Blood causes hemolytic anemia		Cats are more sensitive	Takes a high dose
Grape juice and grape seed extract	None	None	None	None
Auto antifreeze	Kidney	Ethylene glycol	Kidney— crystal formation in the kidneys. Can recover with low dose	Death from kidney failure
Poinsettia	GI tract	Similar to grass	Vomiting Diarrhea	No known deaths
Peanuts, nuts	None	Safe	None but obesity from the fat on nuts	None

Chocolate	GI, pancreatitis, heart, central nervous system	Theobromine toxic doses Milk chocolate toxic dose 1 oz. per lbs. body wt. Semisweet toxic dose 10 oz. per lbs. body wt. Bakers chocolate toxic dose 10 oz. per 9 lbs. body wt.	10 mg/lbs. Vomiting, restlessness, excitement, increased urination, muscle tremors, rapid heart rate	Heart problems at 20–25 mg/ lbs. Seizures start at 25–30 mg/lbs. Death and associated heart problems and pancreatitis
Mushrooms, amanita most common-causing toxicity	Most often GI tract issues	Depends on type of mushroom eaten; not all are toxic	Vomiting, diarrhea, abdominal pain, lethargy	Jaundice (yellow skin and eyeballs) seizures, coma, excessive salivation
Scented candles	No effects; some are allergic to the ingredients of candles	Perfumes and wax	Nausea, diarrhea, and vomiting	No known deaths
Iron overload, drinking rusty water (red color is iron)	Iron overload is a liver problem	Water with iron is not absorbed in doses large enough to cause toxicity	None	None

Lead poisoning from ingestion	Liver and brain from ingestion	Lead	Central nervous system signs and stippling in red cells, anemia, colic, vomiting, blindness, ataxia, muscle spasms	Death
Lead from buckshot and other types of ammunition	Pain and no effect due to the lead in the body—has to be in the digestive tract to cause problems	None	None except for pain from the shot	None except for pain from the shot
Macadamia nuts, acorns, avocados	Muscles	Tannic acid	Weakness, tremors, ulceration of the mouth	Kidney damage
Mistletoe, holly, amaryllis	GI tract, lungs	Resins	Vomiting, diarrhea, depression, tremors, drooling, abdominal pain	Death
Naphthalene or mothballs	GI tract and systemic effects	Naphthalene	Lethargy, weakness, vomiting, diarrhea, abdominal pain	Lack of appetite, seizures, coma, death
Alkaline batteries	GI tract	Alkaline	Necrosis of stomach, esophagus, and mouth	Ruptured organs via burning holes in gut, death

oz = ounces, lbs. = pounds, wt = weight

OH MY GOODNESS! IBUPROFEN

The bad news is that Ibuprofen is one compound that has many animals going to poison centers or the pet's doctor and or to cremation centers since this is not a drug that agrees with pets. In fact, it is a red flag—a *no-no* for pets. This compound is frequently used by people for many reasons and people seem to believe that "it is good for me—and it should be good for my pet."

In reality, this is the most toxic substance reported to poison control due to use in dogs, cats, and ferrets. Ibuprofen in a container seems not to be enough to keep pets from getting into the drug. The coating is a sweet compound; when a pet gets the opportunity to consume this drug, it certainly eats more than their share of the compound.

Ibuprofen blocks necessary enzymes and reduces the body's inflammatory responses. The compound hits a high level between 47–120 minutes, depending on tablet, chewable, or liquid form. The liquid is quickest, and chewable forms are next. If an owner thinks that giving this medication with food is the way to give Ibuprofen, he or she could not be more wrong. The food will indeed slow down the time to obtain peak levels. Peak levels will still be reached, although it will take longer to achieve peak levels. The compound is excreted by the kidneys, and the time for dogs to eliminate one-half of an Ibuprofen (half-life) is about 3.9 to 5.3 hours, which is enough time to do lots of damage. In cats, it is worse because cats lack enzymes to metabolize Ibuprofen, making this compound even worse than aspirin.

There have been people who give Ibuprofen to pets for prolonged periods, which has caused fatal gastric perforations, renal insufficiency, or failure, or impaired liver function. Signs of toxicity in dogs, cats, ferrets, and humans are associated with intestinal, renal, and central nervous system—as well as vomiting, bleeding from the nose, and diarrhea, which can occur within twenty-four hours.

Doses of 10–50 mg per pound (25–125 mg/kg) can cause vomiting, diarrhea, abdominal pain, lethargy, and nausea. Giving a dose of greater than 70 mg per pound (175 mg/kg) will cause all the previous signs—plus bleeding of the intestines, excessive water consumption, excessive urination, scanty urination, uremia, and renal failure.

Greater doses of about 160 mg per pound (400 mg/kg) will also cause seizures, inability to walk correctly, and shock or coma. Mega-overdosing of 240 mg per pound (600 mg/kg), which is the minimum lethal dose in dogs, causes death. This drug should not be used in pets. All of these signs can be in cats at much lower doses; cats are thought to be twice as sensitive to Ibuprofen as dogs due to an inability to secrete the drug. Ferrets are even more sensitive.

TREATMENT
Do not give Ibuprofen to your pets. If you have—and your pet has issues—then this is an emergency for your pet's doctor to handle. The sooner you can get your pet to the emergency clinic, the better chance of getting your pet to pull though. If you use Ibuprofen, you might consider purchasing pet insurance. I'm only kidding—but it is playing with fire.

PREVENTION
This is very simple—do not give Ibuprofen to your pets.

RESPONSE TO POISON EMERGENCIES

Most owners do all they can to keep their pets safe and protect them from hazards. It seems difficult to keep pets away from the bad stuff that causes systemic toxicity. Poison control centers receive thousands of phone calls every year about pets that have gotten to some sort of toxin in the household. Some pet owners are not even aware that things in the household can be toxic, and it comes as complete surprise that the pet buddy is very sick from some toxin it may have obtained in or around the house or in the neighborhood.

The biggest issue with people and emergencies is being able to keep calm and not panic. If you feel your pulse and respiration quicken, slow down, count to ten, and start over. It takes courage to be calm in an emergency, but you can do it. Just say, "If it is to be, it is up to me," over and over and do what you need to do. Just do it.

It might be tempting to toss your pet some leftovers, but you are training the pet to look for more of the same kinds of foods. Alas, your pet finds these foods in the garbage, in the yard, or down the street. A pet without a leash can get into garbage that may have been in the hot sun. Time and hot weather cause bacteria or other toxic compounds that only a buzzard can eat and not get sick, but they can kill a pet.

A low kitchen cabinet door left ajar invites a cat to climb in and consume toxic compounds under the sink. Products under a sink can burn an esophagus all the way to the stomach or kill or make a pet very sick. It is advisable to keep all cabinets secure or locked. Move any toxic compounds under the sink to a safer place where pets and children cannot get into.

There are many foods consumed by people that can be deadly to pets. The list of foods that are toxic is rather lengthy and can be found quickly on a downloadable app on iPhones. The app is provided by "Pet Poison Helpline." Go to the App Store on your iPhone, put "pet poison help" in the search line, and it will pop right up. It is easy to use. You can find any substance you think may be a problem.

The app will allow you to quickly determine what hazard the substance will cause. It will also let you read the signs you can expect as a result of the compound consumed. You can call your veterinarian or a poison control center. I like the app a lot as it is so easy to use; each toxin is listed alphabetically. Touch the compound you are looking up, and a color photo shows the compound or plant so you can see the toxic substance in color. At the top, a yellow line will let you know if the toxin is mild, moderate, or severe. It gives a list of signs that can be observed in the pet. It has a silhouette of the pets it will affect, and there are instructions at the bottom. Each button takes you to a description of signs, instructions, or descriptions of the pet poison help line. Another button you can push will connect you directly to the poison control center. How easy is that? Welcome to the modern age. I believe if you are a pet owner, you should have the app on your cell phone.

Allowing a pet to consume sweets may be creating a toxic hazard. If you happen to have any chocolate candies around the house, make sure they are secured—and do not trust a lid to make it safe. You will be sorry if you do. A small amount of anything is not normally a hazard, but very small amounts around the house can be the last straw for a pet. Even potato chips with salt can be bad for pets (due to the salt).

There are so many toxins that it takes an entire book to cover just a majority of them. Tables 7.2 and 7.3 list the most common and most dangerous toxins.

Table 7.2 *Common Pet Poisons*

Prescription medicine	Insecticides
Veterinary medicines	Rodenticides
Over-the-counter medicines	Plants
Lawn and garden products	Household products, paints, and fire logs
Automotive products	

Table 7.3 *Human Foods Poisonous to Pets*

Chocolate (dark varieties are worst)	Coffee	Alcohol
Avocados	Macadamia nuts	Grapes/raisins
Yeast dough	Xylitol sweeteners	Onions
Garlic	Chives	Raw or uncooked meat
Eggs (egg whites)	Bones	Milk
Salt		

CHAPTER 8

GROWTH AND DEVELOPMENT

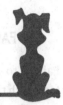

You don't build if for yourself. You know what the
people want—and you build it for them.
—Walt Disney

Growth starts before birth with adequate nutrition of the mamma-to-be. Good nutrition and good health from the mother pet allows the proper nutrients to transfer to the developing fetus. As we all know, nutrition is very essential—and any malnutrition leads to poor health or retarded growth.

Poor nutrition allows for vitamin deficiency that results in abnormal growth and development and brings on slow growth. Homemade diets are often a cause of such deficiencies if the diets are not balanced for vitamins and fats as required by the young or the old to maintain good health.

Many pets that arrive at shelters show the effects of very poor diets. Many animals arrive looking like they came out of a World War II prisoner-of-war camp and are skin and bones. Poor nutrition creates many metabolic diseases that affect hormonal regulations and the genetics of pets. Genetics play an important role in the development of pets. Genetics determine eye color, coat color, rejection of skin grafts, and many other important traits of development. In fact, a quirk of genetics can cause breed changes and even new breeds or abnormalities of development. Breeding of animals can allow for the development of special diseases due to inheritance. In this chapter, we will discuss topics that are associated with growth and development of dogs and cats.

FAILURE TO GROW OR INCREASE BODY SIZE

Failure to grow or increase in size is a rather common phenomenon for which there are many causes. Many factors are complex, and others are rather simple. The factors are too numerous to discuss here, but we will explore three or four of the more-common and less-complex issues. These are the most frequent reasons for failure to increase in body size.

A common cause is being a runt of a litter of kittens or puppies. This phenomenon is genetic and may be a permanent health issue, such as diabetes, congenital heart issues, or other congenital problems. Although the concern may be recognized, many runt causes are not treatable. There are some conditions that might be treatable but require special tests to attempt to rule out a possible treatment plan. More often, there is little that can be done to overcome newborn runt syndromes. The small size does not necessarily mean that the runt of the litter will not be a good pet if all other health issues are within expected limits.

Internal parasites are a common problem that prevents normal growth rates in young animals. Newborn cats and dogs can be born with parasites or obtain parasites through the milk of the mother while nursing. This can be quickly overcome by treating for parasites. Parasite treatment dosages for kittens and puppies can be found in Table 8.1 just after the discussion of prevention.

Nutrition is a common cause of frequent growth retardation. Unfortunately, it is often due to a lack of sufficient food. Many homemade diets lack adequate nutrition. Purchasing poor or cheap pet foods that do not provide the proper nutrients or caloric ingredients for the pet's stage of life is a common issue. Other factors can be blamed too. It is important to mention that feeding an all-meat diet to pets is unhealthy and can result in death, unexplained broken bones, dandruff, and loose stools. There are health issues that are involved with feeding an all-meat diet. The effects of all-meat diets develop slowly. If normal foods or vegetables are fed infrequently, it delays or retards the development of the all-meat syndrome. You are probably aware that some foods cause vomiting and/or loose stools; if so, you need to change the diet to one that is tolerated by the pet.

TREATMENT

The best prevention of this issue is to purchase good, well-balanced pet foods and have routine parasite exams. See parasite treatment for kittens and puppies below.

Caution: Do not use adult doses for kittens or puppies. If you obtain Panacur at other places than a feed store, follow directions on the package.

PREVENTION

Good nutrition is essential with frequent feedings. In a shelter, many skinny animals are admitted—and all they need is to be feed. It is sad but true. Semiannual trips to the pet's doctor are an excellent way to stay on top of growth issues as well as many other diseases that can be prevented by simply having a follow-through program to provide a good preventive medicine program for your pet that you and your veterinarian have agreed upon.

Table 8.1 *Kitten and Puppy Dose by Weight of Fenbendazole (Panacur)*

100 mg per cc solution available at feed stores.
Repeat dose every two weeks and continue until
the newborns are sixteen weeks of age.

Weight (in grams)	Dose in cc (to be given by mouth)
100	0.1
200	0.2
300	0.3
400	0.4
500	0.5
600	0.6
700	0.7
800	0.8
900	0.9
1000	1

EXTRA TOES OF CATS (POLYDACTYLY)

[Polydactyly (poly = many, dactyl = digit, ly = plural therefore polydactyly = many digits pronounced polly- dact- ta- lee)]

The cause of this syndrome is an autosomal dominant trait with variable expressions. This gene dominance has resulted in many cats having extra toes or digits and normally has no problems. Perhaps the most common issue with polydactyly is an occasional failure to trim toenails that become embedded and create pain or infection. On occasion, there are conditions that might create lameness in polydactyl cats. However, this is quite rare. Many people like the extra toes and think they are neat. The findings are much more frequent now—most likely due to mating habits of cats, which have spread this condition through dominant genetics. There is no sex preference, and it is expressed equally in male and female cats.

Normally cats will have five toes on each front foot and four digits on the rear feet. Polydactyl cats will have increased numbers of toes on the front feet, rear feet, or all four feet. At our facility, we see far more front feet with excess toes than rear feet.

Cats with many toes are referred to as "mitten cats," "thumb cats," and "Hemingway cats." Ernest Hemingway kept polydactyly cats, and the name stuck. There is some thought that this trait was brought into the United States from England by shipboard cats. Others argue that the origin was in the United States.

Polydactyly does occur in dogs, but it seems to be rather infrequent—and certainly not anywhere near the numbers in cats. In forty years, I have seen only one dog with polydactyly, and that dog had rather large bones in the feet. Radiography looked similar to cloven-hooved large animals. The dog has no lameness and is very normal. The following are personal photos of a case referred to me:

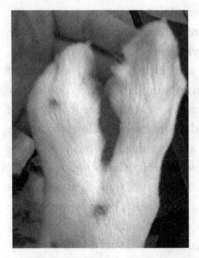 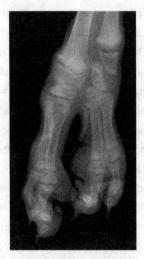

Photo of dog polydactyl **Photo of radiographs of the dog's foot**

WHY ARE ALL MY CALICO CATS FEMALE?

"Why do I have all female calico cats?" This is a frequently asked question. Calico-colored cats tend to be female. Are there any male calico cats? The make calico cat is rare. The so-called calico cat is not a breed of cat; it is a cat with three colors: black, white, and orange. How does it happen? The answer is that the hair coat, like eye colors, is genetic in origin. Orange is one of the three colors that are linked to the X female chromosome. The normal sex of a female is determined by the sex genes; in the normal female, there are two X chromosomes that are commonly designated as XX. You probably remember this from high-school or college biology. The normal male sex genes are one X chromosome and one Y chromosome. The male sex chromosomes are normally designated as XY.

Orange is on the second X chromosome of the female; if a mamma cat happens to have only one female chromosome, or X chromosome, the cat would have what is known as Turner syndrome. The female cat would not be tricolored or be designated as a calico cat. The normal male has only one female or X chromosome—and orange is not present. The fur color has nothing to do with the male chromosome or Y chromosome.

Perhaps you have figured out why there is a male calico cat. If not, you will know shortly. The genetic makeup of the male calico cat is not normal, and the cat has to have a minimum of two X chromosomes. If a male has two female or X chromosomes, the genetic makeup of the male would be XXY. The second X chromosome allows the orange to be exhibited—and therefore is a male calico cat. It is possible for a male to have up to four female sex chromosomes and multiple Y chromosomes. There is a bit more to this syndrome; it also involves dominance, nondominance, and other issues. That is why there are fewer male calico cats. The genetic makeup of the male calico cat is a chance happening of the sex chromosomes that occurs infrequently. An analogy might be throwing dice and expecting six dots to show every time. It just does not happen, and genetics is much more complicated than a single dice roll. As a point of interest, Klinefelter syndrome also occurs in people.

CATS WITH A BROWN EYE AND A BLUE EYE

The brown eye/blue eye comes in two packages. Both are basically genetic, and there is no treatment for either syndrome. We will discuss simple heterochromia iridum or one blue eye and one brown eye in the simplest form of this issue. This syndrome is either genetic or traumatic in origin. Most heterochromia in cats is hereditary. On occasion, it can be the result of disease or trauma. The latter two causes occur in a cat that at one time had both eyes the same color. The disease or trauma results in the iris losing some pigment. Other than the cat having a blue or lighter iris, there is no other medical condition wrong with the cat. It is referred to as *simple heterochromia* because there are no other issues associated with the eye-color difference.

The lighter eye or blue eye is assumed to be the affected eye, and there may be some decrease in size of the iris, but this is often not noticeable. In some, it is rather prominent, and there is contraction of the iris.

Another syndrome associated with brown eye/blue eye is a condition called Waardenburg syndrome. This is a congenital or hereditary condition that may result in deafness or partial deafness associated with the eye-color difference. You might hear that the blue eye side has the deaf ear. Actually it can be either ear—or both ears or neither one. With no deafness, one might consider the condition not to be Waardenburg syndrome and only simple heterochromia.

In people, there is often another issue associated with Waardenburg syndrome. With congenital megacolon (Hirschsprung's disease), a cat does not necessarily have megacolon associated with the blue eye/ brown eye and deafness or partial deafness condition. In fact, megacolon can be a condition disassociated from any eye syndrome and usually is a completely separate issue that is not connected with any other condition. It can be a disease of unknown cause (idiopathic cause).

There are syndromes that can be associated with megacolon. A common sign of megacolon is constipation; if your cat is having normal stools, the cat has a low possibility of having megacolon. Diagnosis of megacolon is best made by your pet's doctor since no one can look at a pet and determine if it has megacolon.

TREATMENT

There is no treatment for simple heterochromia iris or Waardenburg syndrome. If your cat happens to have megacolon from any cause, it will normally require surgery. The procedure is referred to as a subtotal colectomy, which is the treatment of choice for most cats.

PREVENTION

Since these syndromes are genetic, do not breed your cat. There is nothing else you can do for prevention.

MISSING TESTICLE (CRYPTORCHIDISM)

Cryptorchidism is failure of the testicle to descend into the scrotum as a developmental problem in the male. Cryptorchidism is a common and frequent finding at Orange County Animal Services. In our shelter, I do about 150 surgeries per week. On average there is about two to three dogs and cats, or about 4 percent of the stray population of the dogs and cats in Orange County, Florida, that are afflicted with cryptorchid syndrome. It is reported that this condition affects about 1–2 percent of cats and dogs. This condition may have genetic components of unknown heritable nature. The testes that fail to descend will still produce testosterone and the noncryptorchid testicle is capable of producing normal spermatozoa; it is reported that bilaterally cryptorchid (both testicles missing) male cats are infertile.

If the pet dog or cat is young, it is often wise to wait till six to eight weeks of age because sometimes the undecided testicle will descend. In actual practice, the testicle does not tend to descend, but it is worth a try. All it takes is some time. The most frequent undescended testicle is the one on the right, but it can occur on either side.

TREATMENT

The treatment of choice is removal of both testicles in dogs and cats. Failure to remove undescended testes can result in cancer.

PREVENTION
As this is an inherited condition, any pet with this syndrome should not be bred and should have surgery to remove both testicles.

PREVENTIVE MEDICINE PROGRAM
FOR PUPPIES AND KITTENS

Each veterinarian and owner will have their own ideas and programs for a preventive medicine program for puppies. Each individual should have their input for developing a tailored program that meets both the owner's and the professional's perspective about the main issue to be covered—and when these items are to happen. In fact, some veterinarians will have a preprepared suggested program for you to evaluate and add to or deduct from as you and your veterinarian agree on what is essential for the health of the newborn kittens or puppies. Therefore, the purpose of this discussion is to acquaint the reader with the items to be included with time frames for a good wellness or preventive medicine program for newborn puppies and kittens.

There are five basic components to a puppy or kitten wellness program:

1. Physical exams—each newborn should have a good physical to ensure that it has no congenital issues and is healthy.
2. Internal and external parasite treatment and/or prevention since puppies and kittens can acquire internal and external parasites easily—and some internal parasites are obtained from the mother and can be present at birth. Parasite control is a very important part of the program for the newborn.
3. Newborn vaccination programs—each veterinary practice will have an individual program of vaccines for newborns. We will not elaborate on vaccines since there will be obvious deviations due to cost considerations and preferences of the veterinarians and owners.
4. A heartworm prevention program should be worked out between you and the pet's doctor. Perhaps the area you live

in has mosquito populations during certain parts of the year. However, regardless of the mosquito population, this simple, cost-effective program should be a year-round program. Disease prevention is always cheaper than the alternative, and there is excessive savings when comparing treatment costs to prevention involving heartworm disease.

5. Owner education is necessary. It is important to ask questions of your wellness program provider so you have a good grasp of the how, what, when, and where pertaining to the wellness program for the newborns.

Timing of visits with your veterinarian may vary from one veterinarian to another, but the following are provided as a suggested guideline:

Table 8.2 *Doctor Visits for Puppies and Kittens*

Doctor Visit	Puppies	Kittens
First visit	6–8 weeks of age	8–10 weeks of age
Second visit	12 weeks of age	12–14 weeks of age (last kitten visit)
Third visit	16 weeks of age (last puppy visit)	As needed or as set by wellness program
Subsequent visits	As needed or as set by wellness program	As needed or as set by wellness program

INABILITY TO EXTEND THE PENIS (PHIMOSIS)

This is not a common finding, but it occurs in both cats and dogs. The most common cause is a small prepuce opening, which prevents the penis from being extended. This is more of a problem for the pet if it is to be used for breeding. If there are no issues with urination, often there is no further treatment necessary. However, sometimes urine burn of the penis and prepuce can be a health issue. Also, if the orifice is such that urine spray goes in odd directions, then surgical treatment is necessary to enlarge the prepuce opening.

TREATMENT

Treatment often depends on the intended use of the male. If it will not be used for mating, perhaps no treatment is necessary. However, if this option is chosen, look for urine burn to ensure all is well within the prepuce. If necessary, have surgery to enlarge the prepuce.

PREVENTION

This is normally a congenital condition; there is nothing that one can do to prevent a small opening in the prepuce. Consideration can be given to not breeding the pet due to possible inheritance of the condition.

INABILITY TO RETRACT THE PENIS (PARAPHIMOSIS)

This is not a common occurrence, but I have seen it several times in dogs. I have never seen it in cats, but it does occur. The most common findings have been foreign bodies wrapped around the penis, such as string, rubber bands, or other items, which completely resolve the issue when removed. Another cause can be due to castration surgery sutures that are placed too tightly over the penis; blood circulation can be slowed or cut off, causing an extension of the penis. If this happens, all that is necessary is to cut the suture that is causing the problem. This will resolve the problem. The most common cause of inability to retract is a dog that has just finished mating; the penis is still swollen, but this will resolve on its own without any treatment. This is often due to a small opening in the end of the prepuce.

If the penis is not necrotic, then removal of any foreign bodies and sutures that may cause penis extension will resolve the problem. However, if the penis is so swollen that it will not retract into the prepuce, then an ointment needs to be applied to the prepuce—and the prepuce must be pulled over the penis. If the penis is black and not easily treated, then surgery to redirect the urine flow may be necessary.

There is a syndrome in which dogs will bite at body parts. Sometimes a dog will mutilate the penis by continually biting at it. To date, there is little that can be done to prevent or treat this type of problem. A surgical procedure that directs the discharge of urine out the back of the dog might be helpful.

TREATMENT

If foreign bodies are involved, they need to be removed. If the damage is severe enough, surgery to redirect urine flow may be helpful.

PREVENTION

Preventing foreign bodies from getting into the prepuce will eliminate many problems. Always provide supervision when the pet is outside.

Table 8.3 *Dog and Cat Ages versus Human Ages*

Animal Ages	Cats Human Years	Dogs under 20 lbs. Weight Human Years	Dogs 20–50 lbs. Weight Human Years	Dogs 50–90 lbs. Weight Human Years	Dogs over 90 lbs. Weight Human Years
1	15	15	15	14	12
2	24	23	24	22	20
3	28	28	29	31	39
4	32	33	34	38	49
5	36	38	39	45	59
6	40	42	44	52	69
7	44	46	49	59	79
8	48	50	54	66	89
9	52	54	59	73	99
10	56	58	64	80	109
11	60	62	69	87	119
12	64	66	74	94	
13	68	70	79	101	
14	72	74	84	108	
15	76	78	89	115	
16	80	82	94		
17	84	86	99		
18	88	90	104		
19	92	94	109		
20	96	98	113		

CHAPTER 9

PUPPIES AND KITTENS

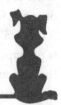

It matters not what someone is born, but what they grow to be.
—J. K. Rowling

Before breeding female dogs or cats, it is best to obtain all the necessary vaccinations. Most vaccines will not affect fetal development, but it is best to immunize early. Dogs and cats are often infested with internal parasites; therefore, treatment for parasites prior to breeding is best and may prevent infections of internal parasites in the newborns. Young animals are most susceptible to disease; attention needs to be given to good nutrition and cleanliness of the breeding and birthing areas.

Normal gestation is about 61–65 days for dogs and 64–66 days for cats. Implanting in the uterus occurs in dogs at about eighteen days and about fourteen days in cats. There can be small swelling at about twenty-one days. Fetal growth is fast, and the fetus diameter doubles about every seven days. At about 35–38 days, palpation becomes difficult until late pregnancy. In this chapter, we will discuss birth and health issues that need attention, and we provide some treatment guidelines for newborns.

NEWBORNS

When dealing with newborn puppies or kittens, it is important to keep track of the litter by identifying each young one so that records can be made for each newborn. One should have a gram scale available. A diet scale that records weight in gram units with a bowl on the top is perhaps the best tool for this purpose; newborns can be placed in the dish and weighed. Failure to gain weight as a newborn is a sign of declining health.

Newborn weights in puppies can vary by breed. The following chart shows weight ranges for size of breed.

Table 9.1 *Newborn Weights in Grams*

Dog Breed Sizes	Weight in Grams
Toy breeds	100–400
Medium-sized breeds	200–300
Large breeds	400–500
Giant breeds	In excess of 700

Puppies generally double their weight by ten or twelve days. Kittens of all breeds normally weigh about one hundred grams plus or minus about ten grams. Kittens often double their weights in about two weeks.

After obtaining weights, other vital signs can be taken and recorded (see pages at back of this book for recording data), such as temperature, pulse or heart rate, and respiration rates. The heart rates are expected to be over 200 beats per minute. Respiration rates of plus or minus fifteen to thirty respirations per minute in both kittens and puppies is the expected range.

There are other diseases that are quite common for newborns in which the stage is set for infections to occur. The main purpose of this topic of discussion is to alert the reader about potential or possible infections. If the mother dog or cat has had hookworms at the time of parturition, then the puppies and kittens can become infected by skin penetration of the hookworm parasites.

Puppies can also obtain hookworms from the milk of the mother during nursing. Thus the stage is set for auto-exposure infections of both puppies and kittens. Roundworms can infect puppies due to what is known as *transplacental infection* and can be born with roundworms, which can be diagnosed in the intestines within one week of birth. Kittens can obtain roundworm infections from the mother's milk since the parasite eggs are also passed in the mother's milk.

It is important that sanitation be maintained for the young, and it is important that all family members know that these parasites (hookworms and roundworms) are infectious to people. Proper care should be taught to all young children handling puppies and kittens to prevent family members from becoming infected with hookworms or roundworms.

There are other newborn diseases, such as fleas. Fleas eat tapeworm eggs; when newborns bite at and swallow fleas, they become infected with tapeworms. I have seen young kittens so infested that they vomit tapeworms. Flea control is important in newborns. Lack of flea control creates heavy infestations of tapeworms in pets; stay on top of flea control for all newborns.

TREATMENT

Treat the worms with just one medicine. Fenbendazole (Panacur) is available at pet stores or feed stores. If purchased at pet stores, follow directions on the package. Table 9.3 is provided for those who purchase Panacur (Fenbendazole) 100 mg/cc Panacur at feed stores. It is important that repeat deworming continue until sixteen weeks of age. Parasites migrate in the body, and the worm medication only treats parasites in the intestines. Do not use adult doses for puppies or kittens.

FOUR WEEKS OF AGE

Newborns sleep and nurse frequently; these behaviors are very normal. Body weight changes are very important to monitor to ensure good health. A failure to gain weight in a few days is abnormal. Lack of weight gain is an early sign of disease in newborns. Body weight should be monitored starting at birth, at twelve hours of age, and daily for the first two weeks.

Identification of the young can be an issue, but it is easy to use characteristic coloring or markings with markers, collars, or ribbons of different colors—or your own ideas—as long as you can identify the same one for several weeks. You can record weight gain or loss on the back pages of this book. You need to note if there are gains or losses since failure to gain weight is often the first sign of illness in a newborn kitten or puppy.

Gram diet scales are cheap and easily available many stores. The weighing container on the top of the scales will help to keep the young from falling off the scales—and make it easier to get the correct weight of the young ones.

Table 9.2 Normal Standards for Kittens and Puppies

Criteria	Normal Standard	Notes
Kitten Puppy medium breeds large breeds giant breeds	100 grams +/- 10 grams 100 grams +/- 10 grams 200–300 grams 400–500 grams 700+ grams	Weights double in kittens: 2 weeks Puppies: 10–12 days
Heart rate C and D	Above 200 beats per minute	C and D = cat and dog
Respiration C and D	15–35 <2 weeks of age	C and D = cat and dog
Body temperature	96–97° F (needs to stay close to the mother)	After 1–2 week increases and by 4 weeks 100° F
Jerking of limbs	Activated sleep	Prevents atrophy
Neuromuscular reflexes	Present at 7 days	
Eyes open	+/- 12–14 days	
Iris is blue gray	Changes to adult color 4–6 weeks	
Normal vision	3–4 weeks	
Flexor tone	Predominates first 4 days, causing comma body positioning of most newborns	
Extensor tone	After 4 days, dominant lies on side with head extended	
Pain perception	Present at birth	
Withdrawal reflexes	Not well developed until 7–14 days	
Start walking	+/- 16 days	
Normal gait	+/- 21 days	

C = cat, D = dog

Table 9.3 *Kitten and Puppy Dose by Weight of Fenbendazole (Panacur)*

100 mg per cc solution available at feed stores.
Repeat dose every two weeks until the
newborn is sixteen weeks old.

Weight (in grams)	Dose in cc (to be given by mouth)
100	0.1
200	0.2
300	0.3
400	0.4
500	0.5
600	0.6
700	0.7
800	0.8
900	0.9
1000	1

Flea treatment can be purchased at pet stores PX and BX military facilities, 1-800 PetMeds, and other online sites. Advantage II does a good job. If large/adult dose containers (blue or red) are purchased and are to be used on animals, use dosages below:

Table 9.4 Flea Medication Dosages

Dogs
Advantage II
Less than 4 weeks of age = 0.1 cc
Between 4–7 weeks of age = 0.2 cc
Dogs greater than 7 weeks
0–10 pounds = 0.4 cc
11–20 pounds = 1.0 cc
21–50 pounds = 2.5 cc
51–100 pounds = 4.0 cc

Cats
Canine Advantage II
Less than 4 weeks of age = 0.1 cc
Between 4–7 weeks of age = 0.2 cc
Cats older than 4–7 weeks
0–9 pounds = 0.4 cc
9+ pounds = 0.8 cc

Activyl is a new flea medication that is available from veterinarians. If you purchase this product in the largest dose, you can dose your pets according to the following chart:

Dogs
Activyl
4–14 pounds = 0.51 cc
14–22 pounds = 0.77 cc
22–44 pounds = 1.54 cc
44–88 pounds = 3.08 cc
88–132 pounds = 4.62 cc

Cats
Activyl
2–9 pounds = 0.51 cc
9 + pounds = 1.03 cc

PREVENTION

Treatment for these parasites should be done before parturition. Mothers should be treated with Fenbendazole on day forty of pregnancy and continue this treatment until fourteen days after giving birth. Use the dosage chart below for adults only. See Table 9.5. Look for your pet's weight to obtain the proper dosage.

Do not overdose!

Table 9.5 *Panacur (Fenbendazole) Dose-by-Weight Chart*

100 mg/cc Panacur [Fenbendazole] Dose-by-Weight Chart
THE FOLLOWING DIRECTIONS ARE FOR NON-PREGNANT ANIMALS
Repeat the dose for three days and then repeat
the three-day treatment in two weeks.
(weight times 25 divided by 100 = dose in cc)

Weight Pounds	Dose cc	Weight Pounds	Dose cc	Weight Pounds	Dose cc	Weight Pounds	Dose cc	Weight Pounds	Dose cc
1	0.25	21	5.25	41	10.25	61	15.25	81	20.25
2	0.50	22	5.50	42	10.50	62	15.50	82	20.50
3	0.75	23	5.75	43	10.75	63	15.75	83	20.75
4	1.0	24	6.0	44	11.00	64	16.0	84	21.0
5	1.25	25	6.25	45	11.25	65	16.25	85	21.25
6	1.50	26	6.50	46	11.50	66	16.50	86	21.50
7	1.75	27	6.75	47	11.75	67	16.75	87	21.75
8	2.0	28	7.0	48	12.0	68	17.0	88	22.0
9	2.25	29	7.25	49	12.25	69	17.25	89	22.25
10	2.50	30	7.50	50	12.50	70	17.50	90	22.50
11	2.75	31	7.75	51	12.75	71	17.75	91	22.75
12	3.00	32	8.0	52	13.0	72	18.0	92	23.0
13	3.25	33	8.25	53	13.25	73	18.25	93	23.25
14	3.50	34	8.50	54	13.50	74	18.50	94	23.50
15	3.75	35	8.75	55	13.75	75	18.75	95	23.75
16	4.00	36	9.0	56	14.0	76	19.0	96	24.0
17	4.25	37	9.25	57	14.25	77	19.25	97	24.25
18	4.50	38	9.50	58	14.50	78	19.50	98	24.50
19	4.75	39	9.75	59	14.75	79	19.75	99	24.75
20	5.00	40	10.0	60	15.0	80	20.0	100	25.0

DOG PARTURITION

The signs that a mamma dog is about to give birth can be very subtle. Signs of impending parturition include: temperature of the mamma dogs will drop to around 99° F (37.2⁰ C), to about 100° F (37.7⁰ C) as temperatures are not constant and can drop in small breeds to about 95° F (35° C); medium-sized dogs around 96.8° F (36° C); and in giant dogs the temp normally falls to about 98.6° F (37° C). The mother dog may show some nesting tendencies during this time. For convenience, birthing is broken down into three stages.

The first stage is often not recognized. There are small uterine contractions and dilation of the cervix. There is vaginal relaxation, and contraction signs are not often noted. The mamma dog may become restless and start panting, rearranging bedding, shivering, and occasional vomiting.

During pregnancy, 50 percent of the fetuses are headfirst, and 50 percent are tailfirst. This change occurs during the first stage of parturition, and the orientation changes where 60–70 percent of the puppies are born headfirst. Changes in orientation leave about 30–40 percent are born tailfirst.

The second stage is when a fetus enters the birth canal—and it ends when the fetus has been delivered. Uterine contractions during this period are strong. The second stage may last up to twenty-four hours. There are three distinct signs that the mamma dog has entered the second stage. If one or more signs are seen, the dog is in second stage of delivery.

- passing of fetal fluids (first water)
- visible abdominal straining
- rectal temperature returning to normal

In a normal delivery, contractions may be weak with infrequent straining up to four hours before giving birth to the first fetus. If the mamma is straining hard during the second stage without producing any pups, this is an indication of birth canal blockage. If there are no pups within forty minutes, help should be sought.

The following are signs that the parturition is not going well and help is needed.

- There is a green discharge, but no puppy is born within four hours. Dark green discharge is an indication that the placenta has separated and is not a good sign. When green is seen, the dog needs help.
- A fetus was born, but no others are within three hours.
- She has weak, irregular straining for more than four hours.
- She has strong straining for more than thirty minutes.
- More than four hours have passed since the last puppy.
- She has been in the second stage of labor for more than twelve hours.

The third stage is expulsion of the placenta (usually within fifteen minutes after the delivery of each fetus). Discharges can often be seen up to three weeks after delivery. The greatest discharge is normally during the first week.

If any of the following signs are noted post-parturition, help should be sought:

- All placentas have not been passed within six hours. This may be difficult to determine as mamma dog may have eaten some. (She should not be allowed to eat more than two.)
- A putrid or foul smell is noted.
- Severe genital hemorrhage.
- The rectal temperature is higher than 101.3 (39.5 C).
- The general condition of the mamma dog is abnormal.
- The general condition of the pups is abnormal.

The normal interval between births in uncomplicated births is about 5–120 minutes. If giving birth to a large litter, the mamma dog may rest for about two hours before resuming the birthing process. Parturition is usually completed within six hours of the onset of second-stage labor. It can last up to twelve hours. It should never be allowed to go twenty-four hours because of risk to the mamma dog and the puppies.

CAT PARTURITION

Cats normally do not have anywhere close to the number of issues that dogs do when it comes to birth of the young. Nutrition during pregnancy is important, but the overpopulation of feral cats might make you think it is not so necessary. However, we can ensure that healthy mamma cats (so-called queens) will birth healthy kittens. There is no way to know the death rates of feral cats, but feral queens produce lots of young. Many feral cats are fed by people, and this helps sustain the feral cat population.

For the pet queen, it is suggested that a premium commercial kitten diet be fed free choice until the fourth week of gestation. From four weeks on, the energy requirements increase—and there may be a need to increase the amounts. However, if the cat is not eating all that is given, do not waste food by putting more in the bowl. From six weeks of pregnancy, energy requirements can double. Do not get carried away and overfeed a pregnant cat.

It is ideal that all vaccines for the queen are given before pregnancy. It is prudent to remember that some drugs given during pregnancy can affect the fetus.

The parturition of queens can be from four to forty-eight hours with an average of around sixteen hours. There are some variations with different breeds of cats, but all take about the same amount of hours. Kittens may be born headfirst or tailfirst, and this is very normal birthing for cats. The variation in time between births of kittens makes it difficult to determine if the cat is having issues or just a normal birthing. An issue for dogs and cats is making a ringside show out of the birthing process. Seclusion and quiet is preferred by dogs and cats at the time of parturition.

Many pets in the process of having young have been brought to the clinic because the birth process was not progressing as expected. The mamma was placed in a cage, and a cloth was placed over the cage. The lights were turned off to allow private, quiet birthing to progress normally without any issues. A check every now and then was made to ensure that all was going well. A C-section was never necessary. This does not mean that C-sections are not needed. There are times when they are absolutely necessary.

Difficult births in cats are rare, but they happen. If the cat is still in the birthing process at forty-eight hours, it should be seen for treatment or to ensure that all is well with the queen.

TREATMENT

I work in a shelter where there have been thousands of kittens born without any issues. In eight years, there have been no difficult births noted in queens. All have been fed normal Science Diet cat food with no special supplementation. Quiet and seclusion are the secret to quick and normal delivery with occasional checks of the queen and newborn over the period of birthing.

PREVENTION

Immunizing all cats prior to pregnancy is preferred. Immunizations help ensure that cats are healthy for the pregnancy. At the shelter, we do thousands of cat spays. In the eight years of my employment at the shelter, two cats had ectopic pregnancies with the fetus in the abdominal cavity. At time of entry for surgery, there were no indications that the cats had any health issues—and certainly no ectopic pregnancy was expected. The fetus in the abdomen was badly decomposed and bound in the omentum of the abdomen. (Omentum is a fat-looking, lacy membrane in the abdomen attached to the stomach with a function to wall off infections in the abdomen).

SIGNS OF DIFFICULT BIRTH (DYSTOCIA)

This discussion is for alerting you to the signs of a difficult delivery that needs help. One needs to know when you had better seek help for the pet that is in the process of delivering a newborn. Difficult birth is more common in small-breed dogs, brachycephalic breeds, and miniature breeds, but any dog or cat is a candidate for a difficult birth process.

Stage one of delivery is when the temperature of the mamma dog has dropped to below 100° F (37.8° C) and has minor contractions. If this stage has been in progress for more than twenty-four hours, if the contractions are visible, or the mother is in active labor for more than sixty minutes without a birth, help is needed.

- If the fetal membrane has been noted for fifteen minutes or longer and no birth has occurred, there is normally a problem—and mamma needs help.
- If there is greater than four hours between deliveries, the mamma needs help. A newborn may be blocking the birth canal.
- If the delivery is taking more than twenty-four hours for puppies or thirty-six hours for kittens, there is a need for help.
- If there are weak and/or infrequent labor contractions, there is a need for help.
- If there is a green discharge, there is a need for help.
- If there is excessive vaginal bleeding or discharge, the pet needs help.
- If breeding dates are known or you suspect that the mamma has gone for greater than seventy days (and a maximum of seventy-two days), you should suspect the mamma is having problems with delivery. This is way past when the young should have been born.
- If kitten delivery has not occurred within sixty-eight days of the breeding date, help is needed.
- If there are more than fifty-eight days between heat periods, this is a sign of a potential issue that requires investigation to ensure that the pet is doing okay.

TREATMENT

In each case mentioned above, there is a need for the mamma's doctor to intervene and aid with the problem. Delays may result in the death of the mother pet and the young.

PREVENTION

There is little one can do to prevent difficult birth since it often develops in the process of giving birth.

DETERMINING THE SEX OF CATS

When presented for surgery, many owners have no idea what the sex of the cat is. This may seem strange, but it is one of the most frequently asked questions. All one has to do is look, but that is not what happens. We will discuss how you can determine the sex of your cat. It is not rocket science.

There are two issues that are involved in the sexing of cats—whether the male is intact or has been neutered. We will discuss both issues. One might think that this is an issue for young kittens, but it's more often an unknown for adult cats.

Gently lift the tail and look at the spacing between the anus and sex organs (genitalia). Male cats have a greater distance between the anus and the sex organs or genitalia (about 0.5 inches, 1.27 cm apart). The penis is normally out of sight, but it will have the appearance of a hole and not a slit.

If the cat is a female, the anus and vagina opening are closer together or almost right next to each other. The vaginal opening looks more like a slit than a round hole. If looking at a male cat that has been neutered, the testicles will be absent—and male cats can look similar to female cats. Gently lift the tail and look at the spacing between the anus and the sex organs (genitalia).

Male cats that have been neutered have a little more than 1 inch or 2.5 centimeters between the anus and the genitalia.

If the cat is female, the vaginal opening and the anus are almost next to each other. The genitalia will have a slit-like appearance.

HOW TO DETERMINE SEX OF A CAT

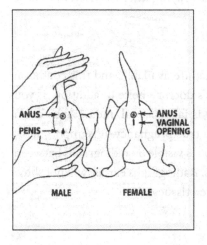

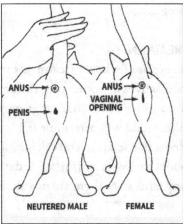

FALSE PREGNANCY

False pregnancy is common in dogs and seldom occurs in cats. Many have false pregnancy and show signs of being pregnant. In false pregnancy, pets show signs of pregnancy and display maternal behavior and physical signs of pregnancy. False pregnancy can occur at any age and does not affect any future breeding.

Signs may include behavioral changes, such as nesting, mothering activity, and self-nursing. There may be abdominal distention and mammary gland enlargement. The false pregnant pet may also have vomiting, depression, anorexia, and no interest in eating. On occasion, the pet may also show signs of labor. Stimulation of mammary glands should be minimized to limit the hormones that stimulate lactation.

False pregnancy is not thought to be influenced by any previous pregnancy, and it does not predispose the mamma pet to other reproductive diseases. False pregnancy is a normal phenomenon, and there is no association between false pregnancy and reproductive abnormalities. If spaying of the pet is being considered, it should not be done during a false pregnancy. If spaying is completed during false pregnancy, it often results in a need to medically treat the pet for false pregnancy. There are no problems spaying after completion of false pregnancy.

TREATMENT

There are no home treatments that are available, and this condition normally will not require the pet's doctor's help. In addition, if you are unsure if the false pregnancy is false or real, radiographs or an ultrasound will determine if it is a true pregnancy. It is important to know that fetal skeletal calcification is visible on radiographs between about thirty-six and forty-five days. Radiographs earlier will not show any fetus since there are no calcified tissues.

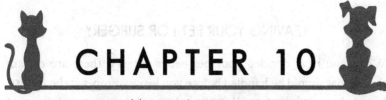

CHAPTER 10

DOES MY PET NEED SURGERY?

Life is like a box of chocolates. You never know what you're gonna get.
—Forrest Gump

Surgery for any pet is always a stressful event. The animal has to go through a lot of steps before ever getting to a surgery room.

The idea of surgery on your pet is a stress on you. The pet has to be left in a facility for blood work and be placed in a cage. All kinds of surgery—from cosmetic to lifesaving—and each comes with a certain amount of risk for the patient.

Whenever an animal goes under anesthesia, there is a risk of the heart reacting to the anesthesia or all of the capillary beds opening up at once, which essentially removes blood circulation from the body within seconds. Of course, every possible safety measure is taken to preclude traumatic events from occurring. Thousands of dollars are spent on obtaining the best and most up-to-date equipment for the safety of a pet in surgery. Unfortunately, bad stuff still occurs, and there is absolutely nothing that is more depressing to a veterinary staff or owners than an unexpected death related to surgery.

We all know that the surgery is necessary—or the pet would not be present for surgery in the first place. Many, many, many, surgeries are extremely successful, and that is the goal. We all want the very best for the patient—and a happy result for the client and pet and success is always the goal of every hospital. With this in mind, we will discuss some surgery issues and perhaps some that may not even need to be done. The final decision on any surgery is always between you and the pet's doctor. There are no exceptions to this rule.

LEAVING YOUR PET FOR SURGERY

When you have decided your pet needs surgery, there are certain things that should be handled before you leave your pet at the facility. It must be noted that not all facilities have all the suggested points of concern to be covered before you leave your pet off for surgery of any kind. Normally the recommendations for surgery will be based on the established standards of care for the hospital or clinic, and each will most likely have a specified treatment plan.

The following checklist will give you a good understanding of the surgery, costs, follow-up plans, and other essentials. If you cannot remember this checklist, take it with you to the pet's doctor's offices. Stay tuned for what you need to know when you leave the veterinary office:

1. Discuss any treatment plans and options for your pet so you understand the charges and any decisions you need to make before or after the surgery.

2. Make sure you understand what is being said. If the doctor uses terms you do not understand about diagnostics or medications, get it clarified on the spot. Do not wait, because you may forget.

3. The doctor should explain preanesthetic, diagnostics, anesthetic monitoring protocols (can be the difference between life and death), pain control procedures, hospitalizations, and nursing care standards. If not covered, you should ask about these issues and determine if there are any additional charges for these services.

4. Make sure the doctor explains the surgery so you understand what is going to occur. Feel free to ask questions about

anesthesia, surgical procedures, follow-up exams, medications, and any other concerns you might have about the surgery. It is important that you know; ask questions and let your concerns be known.

5. You should discuss and accept all *foreseeable* charges, and each should be explained. You should accept these charges; if it makes you feel more comfortable, get it in writing. Ask what unforeseeable things might occur—and what charges can be expected if they do. You do not want any financial surprises; make sure you understand all expected charges clearly.

6. You need to know what presurgical procedures to follow to get your pet ready for surgery. This includes such things as not feeding the pet before surgery since it can cause surgery delays.

7. Ask about shaving the hair so you know what to expect when you pick up your pet. Will they trim your pet's nails for you?

8. If presurgery blood work is to be done, what type will be required? Most places will do a complete blood count, blood chemistry, and heartworm test. When does it need to be done? Most will want this information prior to the surgery date so proper decisions can be made for the surgery. If necessary, schedule a visit to the pet's doctor for the blood work.

9. Will the hospital or clinic call a few days ahead of time to confirm the surgery appointment? At our facility, more than 50 percent of dog owners miss their surgery dates. Do not be one of these people. Be prompt.

10. Tell the doctor or person collecting information how you want to be contacted and leave proper phone numbers where you can be contacted. It is important that a proper phone number is given. Contacts can get mixed up. It is an important step; make sure it is correct. Most will want to contact you after the surgery is complete to let you know how your pet is doing. Many will make follow-up calls several days after the surgery.

11. Determine the expected discharge date so you can plan on picking up your pet on time. If you leave your pet for

longer than planned, you will most likely be charged extra for nursing care, boarding, feeding, etc. Pick up your pet on time or expect extra charges.

12. If there is a discharge appointment, be sure to pick up your pet on time. It will save you money.

13. If medications are to be dispensed, be sure to pick them up at time of discharge. You do not want an extra trip to the doctor's office to pick up medicine. It has happened so many times. When you get the medicines, put them in your pocket or purse. Be sure not to leave them on the counter; it happens all too often.

PREVENTION

Some surgeries do not come with a preventive program, such as planned cosmetic surgeries or spaying or neutering. Traumatic surgeries can be prevented if one accompanies pets outside. Do not let pets roam unattended. Unattended pets account for approximately 98 percent of traumatic events; the other 2 percent involve toxic substances and other causes.

ANAL OR RECTAL PROLAPSE

Anal prolapse seems to most commonly occur in young cats at our clinic. However, it occurs in animals of all ages due to many different causes.

What is an anal or rectal prolapse? It is a partial or completed exposure of the large intestine through the anal orifice to outside of the body. It is often red to red-brown in color; the intestinal mucosa that is exposed to the outside world can be minimal or extensive. Just about anything can cause involuntary straining (tenesmus). Tenesmus is a painful spasm of the anal sphincter that causes an urgent desire to evacuate the bowels or bladder or anything that causes involuntary straining. Since it is easier to say tenesmus than to repeat a two-sentence definition, I will henceforth use the word tenesmus.

The causes of tenesmus are many, but one of the common causes of rectal prolapse—and the easiest to prevent—is caused by internal parasites. At our clinic, the most common parasites causing this condition have been tapeworms in cats and whipworms in dogs. The causes of tenesmus include inflammations of the distal colon, colonic tumors, anal tumors, foreign bodies, constipation, hernias of the anal area, parasites, and difficult births. Some you can prevent; others are endemic or not controllable by you. The purpose of this discussion is to identify those things you can control. We hope the infections, tumors, and other causes do not happen. The goal of this discussion is to prevent prolapse.

Parasite control is extremely easy since you can purchase Panacur at pet stores or feed stores. If you purchase Panacur from a feed store, purchase 100 mg per cc or per ml (milliliter). Use Table 10.1 for your pet's dose of Panacur. All you need to know is the weight of your dog or cat and look up the dose by weight in the chart.

The Panacur will treat all the parasites in the intestines. Since parasites have a migration phase, you only treat those in the intestinal tract—and must repeat the dose in two weeks. After the second three-day treatment, wait two weeks before getting a fecal run to make sure you have treated all the parasites. Get the dose from the chart, treat for three days, and repeat the three-day treatment in two weeks.

TREATMENT

Unfortunately, a hernia is a job for your pet's doctor since anesthesia and surgery will be required. If it is a small prolapse, the repair will most likely be a simple purse-string surgery. If large, it might need major surgery. Give the Panacur dose for three days—and repeat the three-day treatment in two weeks followed in two weeks by a fecal exam.

PREVENTION

The prevention that you can most influence is preventing internal parasites, which is very simple. It can be done on a routine basis once or twice a year. Overfeeding of bones often causes impacted intestines, resulting in constipation, which causes straining or tenesmus in dogs.

I have seen the large intestine so impacted with bones that I thought I would need a stick of dynamite to free the dog of its constipation. Only kidding—please do not dynamite your pet.

Table 10.1 *Panacur (Fenbendazole) Dose-by-Weight Chart*

100 mg/cc Panacur [Fenbendazole] Dose-by-Weight Chart
Repeat the dose for three days and then repeat
the three-day treatment in two weeks.
(weight times 25 divided by 100 = dose in cc)

Weight Pounds	Dose cc	Weight Pounds	Dose cc	Weight Pounds	Dose cc	Weight Pounds	Dose cc	Weight Pounds	Dose cc
1	0.25	21	5.25	41	10.25	61	15.25	81	20.25
2	0.50	22	5.50	42	10.50	62	15.50	82	20.50
3	0.75	23	5.75	43	10.75	63	15.75	83	20.75
4	1.0	24	6.0	44	11.00	64	16.0	84	21.0
5	1.25	25	6.25	45	11.25	65	16.25	85	21.25
6	1.50	26	6.50	46	11.50	66	16.50	86	21.50
7	1.75	27	6.75	47	11.75	67	16.75	87	21.75
8	2.0	28	7.0	48	12.0	68	17.0	88	22.0
9	2.25	29	7.25	49	12.25	69	17.25	89	22.25
10	2.50	30	7.50	50	12.50	70	17.50	90	22.50
11	2.75	31	7.75	51	12.75	71	17.75	91	22.75
12	3.00	32	8.0	52	13.0	72	18.0	92	23.0
13	3.25	33	8.25	53	13.25	73	18.25	93	23.25
14	3.50	34	8.50	54	13.50	74	18.50	94	23.50
15	3.75	35	8.75	55	13.75	75	18.75	95	23.75
16	4.00	36	9.0	56	14.0	76	19.0	96	24.0
17	4.25	37	9.25	57	14.25	77	19.25	97	24.25
18	4.50	38	9.50	58	14.50	78	19.50	98	24.50
19	4.75	39	9.75	59	14.75	79	19.75	99	24.75
20	5.00	40	10.0	60	15.0	80	20.0	100	25.0

UMBILICAL HERNIA

An umbilical hernia, or a protrusion at what we normally call a belly button, is due to a hole in the abdominal cavity at the location of the abdomen umbilicus or belly button. It can be small or large.

The size of hole in the abdomen dictates the size of the hernia. If the hole is large, organs can be involved in the hernia. Most often, this type of congenital finding is small and only involves a bit of fat within the hernia. The issue becomes a question of whether the pet needs a surgical correction. Some do—and some do not. It is always best to have a hernia repaired.

If pennies and nickels are an issue, you can try to reduce the hernia by pushing the expelled abdominal contents back into the abdomen. Do not be a gorilla when pushing on the hernia; be gentle. The resistance is normally attachments of fat to the sides of the hole in the abdomen, which prevents you from returning the contents to the abdominal cavity. If the hernia is small and the herniated mass cannot be easily pushed back into the abdomen, surgery is usually not required. If the herniated fat or other organs can be replaced into the abdomen, this is often a sign that surgery is a good idea.

If the contents can be pushed back into the abdomen, then the size of the opening can often be determined by placing a finger— or more—in the hole. Be gentle doing this; all you are trying to do is determine the size of the hole. If a real small hole is found, surgery might not be necessary. However, if a large hole is palpated after pushing the contents back into the abdomen, surgery becomes important since organs could escape and become strangulated in the hernia and kill your pet.

If you feel uncomfortable dealing with an umbilical hernia issue, the pet's doctor can help you to decide the best actions to be taken. The doctor has experience dealing with these issues and will be able to give you a good answer to determine if the pet needs surgery.

TREATMENT

The treatment for a hernia is surgical correction. However, many pets have small hernias that do not require surgery. Just because there is a small hernia does not mean that surgery is necessary.

PREVENTION

Since an umbilical hernia is a congenital condition and is present at birth, there is no known prevention that can be performed.

INFECTIONS AROUND THE ANUS (PERIANAL FISTULA)

Infected or draining infectious tracts around the anus of some dogs are a chronic condition that requires surgery. An antibiotic without surgery normally is not effective. There may be perianal adenomas (adenoma is a benign tumor of a glandular structure) associated with the infection. Adenomas in the anal and genital area (perianal region) can be solitary or multiple and can be slow, round, lobular, hard, and variable in size. This is a painful area for the dog and may be a reason for the pet to bite at the area.

German shepherds and Irish setters are more prone to anal fistulas, but that does not exempt any breed from this disease. Sometimes neutering will reduce the incidence of this condition. However, in older dogs, neutering does not seem to be effective in preventing this disease. The cause of this disease is not well defined, but several theories exist. It may be associated with colitis or poor ventilation of the area due to a low tail or a broad tail—and there may be a higher density of sweat glands in the area of the anus.

TREATMENT

Treatment is surgery; any other treatment seems to be a waste of effort and money. There is a risk associated with this corrective surgery; if the anal sphincter muscle is destroyed, the dog will have issues with defecation.

A competent veterinary surgeon will not normally have any problems completing this type of surgery. It is important that all infected materials are surgically removed to prevent any reoccurrence.

This was one of my very first surgeries after graduating from veterinary college.

PREVENTION

The condition is a rather spontaneous occurrence, and there is no special preventive program for anal fistulas. If the problem is identified early, a quick response to treatment might ward off the worst cases of anal fistulas.

CAT TOES TURNED UNDER (TENDON CONTRACTURE)

Some cats have problem tendons on the back side of the leg that contract or become somewhat shorter, which causes the toes to turn down and point backward. It makes the foot look as if the cat is trying to have paw grip or form a fist. This is a frequent finding in some litters of kittens that have the hind feet turned under due to tendon contraction.

The good news for these kittens is that the condition tends to resolve once the kittens become ambulatory. The bad news is the cause of the kitten toes to be turned under is not known. The problem is that owners do not know that most kittens will overcome this issue and may euthanize these kittens due to the tendon contracture—and this tends not to be necessary.

Adult cats may develop tendon contractures—most commonly due to trauma. Adult cats may develop tendon contracture of the front feet for unknown reasons. There are two presentations of this condition in adult cats—minor and advanced cases.

TREATMENT

The best treatment for minor tendon contractions is to provide stretching exercises for the cat's front feet and splinting the feet in a correct position. Advanced tendon contractions may require surgery. Unfortunately, you cannot look at the feet and determine if conservative treatment will be effective. If it is tried and fails, it is time for surgery.

PREVENTION

Idiopathic or unknown causes of tendon contracture cannot be programmed to prevent the tendons from contracting since the stimulus of the contraction is unknown. Adult traumatic events may be prevented by looking around the house and removing potential trauma locations you might identify. This sounds easy, but it may not be as obvious when you look around for possible ways your cat might get hurt.

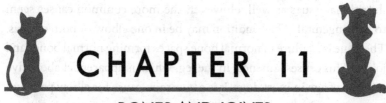

CHAPTER 11

BONES AND JOINTS

You only live once, but if you do it right, once is enough.
—Mae West

Bone and joint injuries are almost always the result of lack of pet supervision outside. The major cause is a pet being hit by a car or HBC (hit by car). Many traumas results from cars. Skin wounds from being dragged along the road happen from meetings with cars. Bad burns, most often on the back, come from exhaust pipes.

By looking at a bone break, it is often easy to tell that the dog was attempting to avoid the car—and received a beautiful spiral fracture. The bad news for owners is that some meetings of dogs or cats with cars result in dead pets or very expensive surgeries.

There are some issues that occur because of non-trauma or congenital issues. e.g. missing ribs, mussle diseases and others. These tend to be developmental, such an elbow dysplasia, which is a lack of proper union of bones. Hip dysplasia is a slow-developing hip joint issue. There have been volumes and volumes written on bone trauma—from how to fix bones to proper nutrition for bone healing. In this chapter, we will not even scrape the surface of bone issues, but I cover a couple of very common bone issues in dogs. Cats have the same issues, but they seem to be very rare.

ELBOW DYSPLASIA

Elbow dysplasia is a common occurrence in dogs. This is often a congenital developmental condition and may be associated with nutritional issues as well. However, the more common causes seem to be congenital. The condition may be in one elbow or both elbows. The issue is a failure of normal bone spaces forming normal bones and joints. This causes lameness in the leg, which is apparent at about five months of age in most dogs. It is a common cause for elbow pain and lameness of the front legs.

Diagnosis is made by radiology and shows the failure of normal bone spaces closing together as the pet ages. Lameness is the most common sign, starting at four months, but it can range up to ten months. Signs are often those of degenerative joint disease. It is interesting that many young animals do not show signs. Furthermore, not all patients will show signs—even though they have elbow dysplasia.

Lameness due to elbow dysplasia is often associated with exercise of the dog, which will show lameness after exercise. When palpating the joint with movement, one might notice crepitus or crunching in the joint along with diminished range of motion of the joint.

TREATMENT
Surgery is the preferred treatment. Pain medication may help the pet.

PREVENTION
This is an inherited condition, and the pet should not be bred.

KNEECAP OR PATELLAR LUXATION

Patellar luxation is a common cause of rear leg lameness in small breeds of dogs (but not often in larger breeds). Patellar luxation occurs in cats, but this condition is quite rare. It seems that female dogs are more often found to have luxation patella syndrome to the tune of about 1.5 times more often than male dogs.

With luxation, the patella moves out of the middle of the knee joint up to the side of the knee. When this occurs, your pet may straighten its leg and hop along and then walk normally. What the dog is attempting to do when it straightens the leg is to get the patella to move back into its normal position. The movement of the patella back and forth causes an intermittent lameness, which is often noted by owners. The patella will move in different patterns; some move to the outside of the knee (laterally), to the inside of the knee (medially in 75 percent of cases), or inside and outside the knee joint.

Some patellae are very lax and may be luxated 100 percent of the time, and others pop in and out of joint. This is most often a congenital condition in small breeds. It can occur as a result of a traumatic event, which will allow the patella to be luxated in one or more directions.

Depending on the severity of the joint problem, the animal may need to be restricted. Certainly many dogs have hop-and-walk syndrome and do quite well. It is not unreasonable to expect arthritis in the joint to develop over time, causing the condition to worsen.

TREATMENT
Surgery can correct or improve the luxating patella. Some will reoccur, and relapse is always possible.

PREVENTION
Since this is most often an inherited condition, breeding of affected dogs should not be allowed.

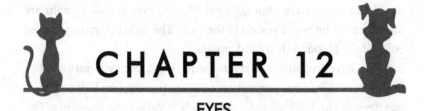

CHAPTER 12

EYES

If a man does his best, what else is there?
—General George S. Patton

Have you ever wondered how an eye sees small items, such as a hair, or mountains and airplanes? The little balls in the head allow the eye to see in color or black and white in day and night, rain, snow, or fog. What a marvel of nature—and how lucky all animals are to have eyes that provide sight to see the world as we know it.

Unfortunately, eyesight can be fleeting due to trauma and aging in dogs and cats. Eye neglect seems to be high on the list of causes of eye deterioration. Some are simple to aid, and others take professional help. The bad news is that once an eye is ruined, there is no replacement. The pet will be blind in that eye or in both eyes.

In this chapter, we discuss eye health for our pets. If there is an eye issue, we want to help the poor pet overcome it. It is my personal and professional belief that eyesight is so precious that eyes should always be seen by professional doctors. Unfortunately, that does not happen frequently, but there are some guidelines.

EYE ANOMALIES NOTED IN A BEAM OF LIGHT

Have you ever wondered why an animal's eyes shine when they get in your headlights or you shine a light at the animal? Why do the eyes of people show up red in photographs? The red eyes in photographs are produced by the blood vessels in the eyes. The light brings out the red color of the blood in the blood vessels.

Pets have two major parts to the back of their eyes (retina). The first part is the dorsal portion that covers the top one-half to three-quarters of the back of the eye, which is called the tapetum. The tapetum has extremely reflective materials within its tissues, and this part of the eye shines back at you when you shine a light at an animal.

The second part is located just below the tapetum, on the back of the eye (retina), where there is a nontapetum area that is normally a dark color and does not reflect light. Many other animals have a reflective tapetum. You might be familiar with teleosts, crocodiles, marsupials, alligators, fruit bats, raccoons, possums, marsupial cows, and horses.

It is thought that the tapetum collects minimal light at night and allows the animal to be able to see better in the dark. Of course, no animal has yet communicated this to anyone to let us know without any reasonable doubt that this is so. However, the best scientific information available tends to support this hypothesis.

BLOOD IN THE EYE (ANTERIOR CHAMBER HYPHEMA)

The causes of blood in the anterior chamber are too many to mention, but they include trauma, fragile or thin-walled blood vessels, clotting disorders, some tumors, and a variety of so-called systemic diseases. We will discuss only very small amounts of blood in the eye—with no repeated bleeding.

To understand the anterior chamber, I will explain a bit of eye anatomy. The clear portion of the eye you see is the cornea. Behind the cornea is the anterior chamber. Behind the anterior chamber is the iris or the portion of the eye that gives color to the eyes.

Due to complexity and various causes of blood in the anterior chamber, the best treatment would be provided by your pet's favorite doctor. It is not necessarily for the treatment of the small amount of blood. The visit to the doctor is to ensure that the cause of the bleeding is not a systemic condition that might continue to bleed into the eye. However, if you are a determined do-it-yourselfer, you can follow these simple steps.

Small amounts of blood released into the anterior chamber will normally resolve due to products secreted by the iris. The result of blood in the anterior chamber may be more traumatic than the bleeding; the blood in the anterior chamber might plug normal drainage parts of the eye and affect vision.

Repeat bleeding is not a good sign for the health of the eye or the pet. There are complex systems that can cause interference with blood-clotting factors and low blood counts to include the all-important platelets. If the pet happens to have glaucoma and recurrent bleeding, it may be a sign of ocular tumors.

TREATMENT
Medications for the treatment of blood in the anterior chamber may not be all that effective, and the best treatment for nonrepeated bleeding and small amounts of blood is time.

PREVENTION
Unfortunately, this condition is considered to be idiopathic, which means it often just happens for no apparent reason or for reasons that cannot be prevented. Therefore, you cannot stop or prevent blood in the anterior chamber from occurring. The best alternative is to take good care of your pet and have a preventive medicine program in effect to ensure your pet maintains its good health. I suggest a visit to your pet's doctor at least two times per year. Prevention is much cheaper than treatment of any kind.

GUNK (EXUDATES) IN THE EYES (KCS)

My personal feeling is that eye issues should be seen by your pet's favorite doctor since eyes are so easily destroyed. Sometimes an eye can look good today and be demolished tomorrow, and it requires special medication to prevent the eye from melting away. Regardless of how bad an eye condition might be, some folks are never going to make an appointment to see a veterinarian. This is the reason for this discussion. One of the most common findings we see in our clinic is dry eyes in dogs—especially the small breed dogs—and the poor buggers have never been treated for the eye problems.

Many phenomena cause dry eyes, including trauma, medicines (primarily sulfa drugs), infections, and idiopathic and congenital issues. The actual cause may not be as important as the need to treat the dry-eye syndrome (more commonly called *keratoconjunctivitis sicca* or *KCS*). The clinical signs of dry eye when you look at your pet's eyes are a thick, often ropy ocular discharge that seems to cling to the eyeball surface and eye dryness. The usual reflective wet surface of the normal eye is absent. The dryness is easy to recognize, and you cannot miss seeing the eye accumulations. You can treat the dryness and accumulation in the eye with over-the-counter medications. The lack of shine on the surface of the eyeball should alert you to the fact that the eye or eyes are dry. Of course, dry eyes are painful to your pet, and moisture applied to the eye/s is always appreciated by your pet.

Signs of KCS can vary, depending on how long the dry eye has been present. It can be chronic, recent, temporary, or permanent. Your pet's doctor has medications (Optimmune or Cyclosporine) that can restart normal eye tear production; this means a trip to the doctor. Optimmune does not always work, but any attempt is better than doing nothing. This drug may require artificial tears on a daily basis. It would be time and money well spent on behalf of your pet.

TREATMENT

My favorite home treatment for dry eyes is GenTel Gel applied to the eye/s for a minimum of four times daily. The time of treatment is not important—just get a minimum of four times a day completed. GenTel Gel is readily available and easy to obtain at grocery stores, pharmacies, Walmart, and many military PX and BX facilities. GenTel Gel is an over-the-counter artificial tear compound. GenTel Gel tends to stay longer in the eye, which is a great benefit.

There are other artificial tear brands; if you cannot find GenTel Gel, use the most viscous artificial tears you can find. GenTel has many different artificial tears of various viscosities—from watery to thick. Unfortunately, dry eyes have to be treated forever—or until the eyes once again produce tears without medication.

While I am on this subject, let's discuss why a minimum of four times a day is important. Let's start with low-viscosity compounds, which are almost like water. If you put this in an eye, it might treat the eye—if we are lucky—for about three minutes. So three minutes times four times a day is a treatment of only twelve minutes in a twenty-four-hour day. That is why I do not like low-viscosity eye compounds. That does not mean I do not use them, but if I have a choice, I will use ointments.

Why is an ointment better? If you put an ointment in an eye, it may last twelve to fifteen minutes in the eye (tears wash it away). Twelve minutes times four times per day equals forty-eight minutes in a twenty-four-hour day—much more than twelve minutes. This does not mean that low-viscosity eye medications do not work, but it explains my bias.

PREVENTION

Many of the causes of dry eye do not have specific things you can do to prevent the condition from occurring—other than tender love and care and good nutrition. There are many breeds that are more prone to dry eye syndrome—West Highland white terriers, American cocker spaniels, bloodhounds, Yorkshire terriers, Boston terriers, Shih Tzus, Samoyeds, Cavalier King Charles spaniels, English bulldogs, miniature schnauzers, Pekingese, poodles, pugs, and English springer spaniels. The majority of cases of dry eyes are idiopathic (occurring without a known cause). Excision of the gland of the third eyelid is a common cause of KCS in dogs.

THIRD EYELID PROTRUSION (CHERRY EYE)

The third eyelid is the pink gizmo in the corner of the eye next to the nose (medial canthus), which is normally not visible. When it is constantly visible, it is a sign that there is some kind of problem that needs attention. You might say it is a red flag.

Causes of the third eyelid being visible are anything that will cause the eyeball to be pulled back into the eyeball socket. Dehydration is one more common causes of third-eyelid protrusion. It is an issue when the pet is dehydrated. The most common pink in the corner of the eye is due to "cherry eye." Other protrusions are due to tumors of the eye or the third eyelid.

Pain in the eye will cause the pet to pull the eye back into the eye socket, which will let the third eyelid protrude. Pain in the eye can be caused by glaucoma, infections of the iris, corneal ulcers, and foreign bodies in the eye or behind the third eyelid.

TREATMENT

Though third-eyelid protrusion can be seen, the issues causing the protrusion are normally beyond the ability of home treatment. It is essential that the pet visits its favorite doctor.

PREVENTION

This is a condition that cannot be predicted. The best plan is to have a good wellness plan set with your pet's doctor.

EYELIDS RUBBING ON THE EYEBALL (ENTROPION)

An eyelid rubbing on the eyeball is a very common finding in dogs and cats. This problem can be very minor with some tearing running down the face, most commonly at the corner of the eye by the nose. It can be really bad if the upper and lower eyelids turn in excessively and rub on the eyeball, creating excessive pain for the pet. In some cases, the eyelids will be so turned in that the eyeball cannot be seen.

There are many causes of eyelids rubbing (entropion) on the eyeball. Skin folds of some animals can result in the eyelids rubbing on the eyeball—or the skin fold will actually rub on the eyeball. Either is very painful for the pet. When an animal experiences pain in an eye, the eye will frequently be pulled back into the eye socket, which can create a condition that allows the eyelid to rub on the eyeball.

If the eyeball is not in its normal position, the eyelid can rub against the eyeball. In my experience, some cases have been so bad that it was thought that extensive corrective surgery would be necessary. However, with topical eye treatment, the eyelids and eyes become normal. This was a huge surprise since the case was really bad. The case was so bad that the eyeball could not be seen; the upper and the lower eyelids were rolled onto the eyeball. This was a learning process; before doing surgery, the eyes should be treated topically. If the eyelid still rubs on the eye, then surgical correction is warranted. One cannot simply look at an eye and know what caused the pain in the eye or that the animal has spastic entropion.

Unfortunately, not all cases will be as easily treated as those that require only topical medications. Most will need surgical correction. Show dogs are often not allowed to have cosmetic surgery. Entropion surgery qualifies as cosmetic surgery.

TREATMENT

Feed stores may have eye medications that you can purchase. In our area, they carry Terramycin ophthalmic ointment. Not all simple medicines in the eye will correct eyelid rubbing (entropion) on the eyeball. Therefore, most will actually require surgical correction. However, it is my belief that eye rubbing should be treated before doing surgery to ensure that the entropion is not the result of spastic pain that can be treated with topical medications.

If eye medicines are not available at the feed store, give 1 (800)-PetMeds a try. They have eye medications. If it takes a prescription, your veterinarian can provide one for you.

PREVENTION

There is not a lot a person can do to prevent eyelids from rubbing on the eyeball. However, one can look at the eyes. If one notices tearing, one needs to carefully look at the eyelids to see if the lids are rubbing on the eyeball. Some very slight rubbing on the eyelid might be seen. This slight rubbing will result in tear production and may stain hair on the face.

Dehydration will cause eyeballs to go back into the eye socket. This contributes to the eyelids rubbing on the eyeballs. A simple personal exam of the eyes can catch small things about to happen. As always, early detection is always good for the pet—and for the cash flow.

DETERMINING BLINDNESS IN PETS

It is far easier to determine blindness in a dog than in a cat. The issue at home with pets is that blindness is normally a slow process. Due to the slow occurrence of blindness, the animal will adjust and know where everything is in the house and will get along very well in the house. Therefore, the owner does not even recognize that the pet is blind. Recognition of blindness in a pet is frequently an accidental finding—unless they happen to take the pet somewhere unfamiliar, such as the clinic or hospital and the pet walks into objects.

A leash can be placed on a dog, and one can deliberately lead a dog to an object; if the dog has very limited vision or is blind, the dog will walk into the object. If the dog avoids the object, it can see—regardless of any reduced vision. Reduced vision or blindness is most often seen in older dogs. Many will have developed mature cataracts or have a disease that causes excessive corneal opacities. If a dog has excessive corneal opacities, sometimes the corneal opacity can be reversed. The dog may see again, although it might have limited eyesight. It may not be reversible.

Cats are more difficult to determine blindness in since they do not jump up and move like dogs do. A cat will certainly adjust to the home environment, and it may be impossible for the owner to even suspect that the cat is blind. Blindness may be due to mature cataracts. This condition seems to be much less frequent in cats than in dogs.

When a cat is in a new environment where it can walk into objects or walls, then a diagnosis of blindness may be in order. The issue for cats is that placing a normal cat that sees okay on the floor does not mean that it will move; it often remains on the floor, especially in a strange environment.

Sometimes the cat may walk as though it is feeling its way along with its front feet. If you wait to see this, you may be in for a long wait—due to the lack of movement of the cat. Dangling an object over the cat or throwing a toy in the air might help—but the cat might sit still. Perhaps the best test is to take the cat, hold it by the chest, and lower it to a table or floor. Since most cats can see they are about to be placed on a surface, they will extend the front legs in preparation. Vision impairment may be an issue, particularly if the cat makes no effort to move its front feet until making contact with the surface.

Sometimes just moving one's hands back and forth in front of the pet will be a way to determine blindness. If a pet can see, it will move its head or its eyes back and forth.

TREATMENT

Unfortunately, there is no treatment for blindness. If the blindness is due to cataracts, it can be overcome. Some veterinary colleges have special equipment that allows them to remove cataracts from small pets and horses. Kansas State University has this ability—and there are others. If you are interested, you can check with a veterinary college to find out if they have the ability to remove cataracts in pets and place a lens for better eye sight.

PREVENTION

Unless there is a specific early diagnosis that can be reversed, there is little or nothing that can be done to prevent blindness in pets.

CHAPTER 13

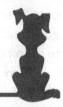

PETS AND TEETH (DENTAL CARE)

Everything has its beauty, but not everyone sees it.
—Confucius

Just a few years ago, teeth in dogs and cats were mostly ignored. There were pets with broken teeth and very dirty teeth. Other than pulling a tooth, not much was done. All of that has changed dramatically, and there is a board specialty devoted to dentistry in veterinary medicine.

Dentistry has moved from the back room to the front room, and veterinary colleges have dedicated facilities for the care of teeth in dogs and cats. It has been shown that good dental care in pets results in less chronic diseases—and longer lives for dogs and cats. In this millennium, you may be taking your pet in for dental care, cleaning, polishing, and perhaps even root canals.

I have pet owners tell me how they brush their pet's teeth. It was not along ago when no one would even consider brushing a pet's teeth. In this chapter, we will discuss dental care, baby teeth, and how to age a pet by teeth.

PET DENTAL CARE

Pet dental care is getting much better attention than in the past—as it should. You know from your own experiences that healthy teeth contribute to overall good health. We want the best for our pets, and good healthy pets are essential for us. Good healthy teeth contribute to the total package of excellent health for pets.

There are many contributing factors that directly affect the teeth of pets. Some are very simple; an example is the kind of foods that are fed to pets. Some foods can cause excessive accumulations on teeth, which contributes to poor tooth health and causes infected gums. This causes extraneous growth of the gum tissues; the pet may bite the tissues, causing a bloody mouth and bleeding gums.

Dirty teeth allow accumulation of bacteria and cause other unhealthy conditions in the mouth, such as periodontal disease, infected gums, bleeding gums, soft tissue loss, and even bone loss. The bone loss allows teeth to become loose and fall out or causes a need to have the teeth pulled. There are many cases of baby or so-called milk teeth not being expelled normally, and the tooth becomes retained.

The milk teeth or baby teeth need to be extracted since they can cause crowding of teeth, resulting in crooked teeth. There are times when the extra teeth cause teeth to point toward the roof of the mouth, which causes pain for the pet due to the malocclusion of the teeth. Soft foods are more likely to cause food particles to accumulate on teeth, and hard dry food tends to clean the tartar from the teeth. Hard food actually helps improve the breath of the pet. I did not say the hard food cleans the teeth—I said the hard or dry foods *tend* to help remove tartar and help the pet's breath improve.

A word of caution is necessary here in reference to feeding hard bones or allowing hard chew toys for dogs. More teeth are broken with these two products than you can imagine, and it can be expensive to have a root canal, tooth fillings, or have infected teeth pulled.

Some clients say, "I was feeding bones before you were born." This may be 100 percent true, but I know what I have treated due to feeding or allowing play with hard bones and chews. The list is lengthy, and you do not want to experience any of them.

TREATMENT

Pet toothbrushes are available to help keep the teeth clean. I have had some clients say the pet likes having their teeth cleaned, and others claim it is a struggle—but they brush the pet's teeth anyway. If you can get a dental scraper, some pets will allow you to scrape tartar from the teeth. Give it a try—and you might be surprised by what you can accomplish with a little persistence.

PREVENTION

Soft foods are more likely to cause food particles to accumulate on teeth, and hard or dry foods *tend* to clean the tartar off the teeth. It is best to start your pet on hard foods rather than changing later. It is a health hazard to feed all-meat diets, which can kill pets.

AGING BY TEETH

Aging by looking at teeth is a ballpark approximation at best, but without a birth date, it is possibly the best way to get an approximate age because there is no other easy way to obtain an age.

At our facility, some ages have been assigned this way, but during surgery, the organs being removed reveal a younger age than the estimate. Of course, if surgery is not being done, there is no way to compare ages with tissues being removed from the body. This observation is easiest to see during a female spay—and is not so for neutering males.

When males are neutered, you can only guess. Even though the exact age cannot be determined by surgery, age by teeth can seem inaccurate. Let's assume an age of three years has been assigned to an animal by observing its teeth. It is easy to detect an age less than a year at surgery. If one looks at belly skin, a determination can be made between really young versus middle age versus old age, but no precise age can be assigned. So we are back to the teeth for getting the best estimate of a pet's age.

There are things that interfere with aging by teeth. If a pet has had good dental care, the pet will have better-looking teeth and will not normally adapt to an age chart very well. If a pet has been a chewer of hard objects or chews on rocks or other object that damage teeth, these behaviors will make the pet's estimated age older than it is.

There are tooth differences between dogs—and even within the same litter. Aging by teeth is the best ballpark method we have to obtain an approximate age of the animal. If you're a horse owner, you know how unreliable age by teeth can be. Having said all that, Table 13.1 is a chart of approximate ages of dogs and cats by observing teeth.

All deciduous (baby teeth) are very close together until two months of age. At two months of age, deciduous teeth spread out. Once all the adult teeth have grown in, age is judged by the amount of tartar on the teeth. When a very thin line of tartar on the molars is seen, age is estimated to be about one to two years of age. With a moderate amount of tartar on the molars, the age is estimated to be about three to five years. Teeth that are covered with tartar—or missing or rotting teeth—places the estimated age to be six to ten years of age. If the pet has had good tooth maintenance, these age estimates mean absolutely nothing.

Table 13.1 *Aging-by-Teeth Chart*

Approximate age	Cats	Dogs
2–4 weeks	Deciduous (baby) teeth coming in	No noticeable tooth growth
3–4 weeks	Deciduous (baby) canine teeth coming in	Deciduous (baby) canine teeth coming in
4–6 weeks	Deciduous lower jaw premolars are coming in	Deciduous incisors and premolars can be seen
8 weeks	All deciduous teeth are in	All deciduous teeth are in
3.5–4 months	Permanent incisors coming in	No permanent tooth growth noted
4–5 months	Permanent canines, premolars, and molars coming in	Permanent incisors coming in; some growth of premolars and molars
5–7 months	All permanent teeth in by 6 months	Permanent canines, premolars and molars coming in, all teeth in by 7 months
1 year	Teeth clean and white	Teeth clean and white
1–2 years	Teeth may appear dull with some tartar build-up and some yellowing on back teeth	Teeth may appear dull with some tartar build-up and some yellowing on back teeth
3–5 years	Teeth show more tartar build-up on all teeth and some tooth wear	Teeth show more tartar build-up on all teeth and some tooth wear
5–10 years	Teeth show increased wear and diseases; pigment may be visible on gums	Teeth show increased wear and diseases
10–15	Teeth are worn and show heavy tartar build-up; some teeth may be missing	Teeth are worn and show heavy tartar build-up; some teeth may be missing

RETAINED BABY (DECIDUOUS) TEETH

Retained baby teeth are a very common issue with young small-breed dogs. A tooth is considered retained when a baby tooth is still present when the permanent replacement tooth starts to erupt. Baby-teeth retention in cats seems to be an infrequent finding, though it can occur in young cats.

There are numerous causes for baby teeth being retained, but the bottom line is that baby teeth should not be present as the animal ages; their presence can cause malocclusion or misdirection of permanent teeth if the baby teeth are not removed. In dogs, permanent tooth eruption starts at three months of age for incisors (front teeth) and about six months for permanent molars (back teeth). Many dogs with retained baby teeth are not recognized as having retained baby teeth until late in life. If there is malocclusion or misdirected permanent teeth, it is too late to remove the baby tooth to allow the permanent tooth to grow in properly. The cause of the smaller-breed dogs retaining baby teeth more than other breeds currently is not known. It may have a genetic connection within the breed line.

TREATMENT
Owners of small-breed dogs can check the mouths of their pets frequently (between three and nine months) to find retained baby teeth. If present, the teeth can be pulled if necessary.

PREVENTION
There is not much one can do to prevent baby teeth from being retained. Since this condition has a genetic connection within the breed, it is desirable that these pets not be bred. This will prevent perpetuation of retained teeth syndrome.

EXCESSIVE SALIVATION (PTYALISM)

This is not a frequent finding, but it does occur in dogs and cats. Not all excessive salivation is a medical issue. Sometimes taking dogs for a ride in a car will cause drooling. Movement of cats in portable cages, particularly on hot days, seems to be a stimulus for excessive salivation. These findings normally subside within hours. We see cat salivation a lot in the shelter, but within hours or the next day, the cat is normal without any treatment.

With persistent salivation, the major cause is the failure of the pet to swallow the saliva that is being produced. One of the first things people think of as a cause is the paralysis of the esophagus to prevent swallowing associated with rabies. This observation keeps lots of people from examining pets that have salivation. This is good and bad since fear of rabies is a good thing to have. The reality of this is that rabies is not common, but other issues are. It could be an oral ulcer or a stuck chicken bone. It could be a bone jammed between teeth or an object stuck in the esophagus.

There are numerous causes of excessive salivating. However, the first thing to do with a pet that has developed persistent salivation is to look into the mouth to see what might be present to produce salivation. Some of the strangest saliva-producing objects are frequently found in the mouth. If foreign bodies are not found in the mouth, look for ulcerations on the gums or cheeks. If you do not find foreign bodies or ulcers in the mouth, it becomes an issue for the pet's doctor.

Some salivation issues require special radiographic procedures. Another cause may be central nervous system problems. Do the simple things before going to the doctor.

TREATMENT

First, separate nondisease salivation (such as transport salivating) from disease salivation. Second, look in the mouth of the pet for ulcers and foreign bodies, which are the most common causes of excessive salivation. A badly infected mouth or ulcers will normally need antibiotics for treatment. Other causes normally require advanced diagnostic techniques by the pet's doctor.

PREVENTION

Good oral health with clean teeth is important for preventing excessive salivation due to trauma. Feeding chicken bones has been, in my experience, the major cause of excessive salivation in dogs.

Oral problems caused by chicken bones appear to be very, very painful and make one feel sorry that the poor pet had to suffer.

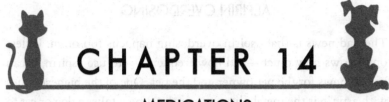

CHAPTER 14

MEDICATIONS

When you get to the end of your rope, tie a knot and hang on.
—Franklin Roosevelt

There are tons of medications: over-the-counter medications, prescription medications, generic and proprietary medications, medications in feed, and others. The issue is not the medication or the type. The proper use of the medication and compliance with the drug is the issue.

Proper storage of medications is so important; children, pets, and others who should not take medications might accidentally suffer the consequences of that drug. Antibiotics are toxins used to kill infectious organisms. Some drugs affect systemic body actions, causing all drugs to have potential toxic effects if not properly used.

Improper storage of veterinary drugs results in thousands of calls to poison control centers every year due to carelessness, improper handling, not putting lids back on, and leaving medications out around pets and children. Not following directions on the label can result in overdosing or insufficient dosing.

It is important to realize that there is a limit to what an owner can do with over-the-counter drugs to aid their pet. In this chapter, we will cover different subjects related to medications that are helpful and harmful if directions are not followed. Remember that medications are for the benefit of your pet—if you follow simple directions and give the medication when you're supposed to, all will be well. *Never* overdose—and always follow directions.

ASPIRIN OVERDOSING

The bad news is that aspirin overdosing happens too often. Unless one knows how much—and how frequently—to use aspirin, it can be bad news for the pet owner and the pet. One of the biggest issues with aspirin is the metabolism rate or the time it takes a dog or cat to eliminate the compound from its body. In cats (depending upon which reference is read), the approximate half-life of aspirin (half-life is the time when half the aspirin dose given will be excreted or metabolized) is 44.6–100 hours. Using the half-life of 44.6 hours and a 100 mg dose aspirin for a cat, in 44.6 hours, 50 mg or half will still be in the cat's body. Because the half-life is so large and so slow, aspirin is a very effective killer of cats.

Signs caused by aspirin are depression or vomiting, which may be tinged with blood. Vomited blood can look like coffee grounds—and has been mistaken for pets eating feces and vomiting it. The trained eye will identify the vomited blood easily. Often the lesions in the stomach will cause bleeding, and you might see red blood in the vomitus. Other signs might include an increased rate of respiration, fever, muscular weakness, unstable standing and walking, coma, and death.

Many other things can cause the same signs. Thus, to know the origin of the problem, the history of aspirin use is necessary to obtain a diagnosis. Of course, you may know you gave aspirin. If you did give aspirin, you know the cause of the signs present. Aspirin will affect the blood of cats—and all of the signs exhibited show that no aspirin products should be given to cats.

TREATMENT

Take your pet to the pet's doctor and tell the doctor what you have done with the aspirin. Do not lie since it is important for the life of your pet. Aspirin can be devastating for your pets, especially for cats. One needs to be darn careful with aspirin.

PREVENTION

To stay on the safe side, do not give aspirin to pets. Only give aspirin as directed by the pet's doctor. Your dog or cat is not a human—and it cannot take aspirin in the dosages or frequency that people do.

ASPIRIN DOSAGES FOR CATS AND DOGS

Aspirin in cats can be deadly, but people reach for aspirin for a cat in pain. Aspirin is not recommended for pets, and many veterinarians will advise clients not to use aspirin. However, not all veterinarians will agree—and some recommend aspirin for dogs and cats.

Pet aspirin is available at pet stores, such as Petco and PetSmart. In this book, we have discussed never using aspirin for pets, but it is known that it will be used anyway. If this is so, it is better to have a dose to recommend than to willy-nilly give aspirin and kill your pet.

For those who insist on using aspirin, the following usage guidelines are provided. Watch for any toxicity that might develop during the aspirin administration and *stop* if you cause vomiting or any other abnormality. Remember that aspirin is not secreted rapidly by a cat. Aspirin doses accumulate in the body due to slow metabolism, and it is extremely easy to create toxicity in dogs and cats.

For cats with pain, elevated temperature, and swelling, use a dose of no more than 10 mg per pound of body weight. Aspirin comes in 81 mg and 325 mg tablets and may need to be cut to get close to the dose needed. Because repeat dosing of aspirin will cause increased concentrations, it is necessary to watch for toxic effects. The following doses are recommended in *Plumb's Veterinary Drug Handbook 7th Edition:*

- Give one "baby" aspirin (81 mg) by mouth every three days. Repeat dose three days later and every third day until not needed. The goal is to give the least amount of aspirin as possible and still have a good response. If every four or five days seems to work, it is better than every three days. This is sometimes possible after one or two doses every three days, and it is definitely worth a try to reduce the dosage of the aspirin.

Or:

- 5 mg per pound (10 mg/kg) by mouth every forty-eight hours.

Cutting an 81 mg aspirin can be very tricky and difficult—especially when trying to get one-eighth of an aspirin. The best one can do is to get close to the calculated dose when cutting tablets.

The following aspirin dosage chart (Table 14.1) is on the light side of aspirin (4.5 mg per pound) of dosing because aspirin and cats are not a good combination. Many cats have been killed with the use of aspirin. Do not let that be your experience. Your veterinarian has much better drugs that work a lot better and faster than aspirin. I strongly suggest that you take your pet to see the pet's doctor for any issue that you feel needs to be treated with aspirin. This aspirin information is provided for those who will not take their pet to see a veterinarian.

Table 14.1 *Aspirin Dosage for Cats*

Use enteric-coated aspirin.
Aspirin 81 MG Tablet

Low dose—give 4.5 mg/pound every seventy-two hours.
High dose—give 4.5 mg/pound every forty-eight hours.
Note: Dosage is approximate due to the need to cut tablets.

Weight Pounds	Low Dose: Tablet or parts of tablet to be given every 72 hours	High Dose: Tablet or parts of tablet to be given every 48 hours	Weight pounds	Low Dose: Tablet or parts of tablet to be given every 72 hours	High Dose: Tablet or parts of tablet to be given every 48 hours
1	Too small	Too small	11	.5 + .12 Or ½ + 1/8	.5 + .12 Or ½ + 1/8
2	Too small	Too small	12	.5 + .12 or ½ + 1/8	.5 + .12 or ½ + 1/8
3	Too small	Too small	13	¾ or .75	½+1/4 or .75
4	¼ or .25	1/4 or .25	14	¾ or .75	½+1/4 or .75
5	1/4 or .25	1/4 or .25	15	¾ + 1/8 or .75 .12	1/2+1/4 + 1/8 or .75 .12
6	¼ + 1/8 or .25 +.12	¼ + 1/8 or .25 +.12	16	¾ + 1/8 Or .75 +.12	¾ + 1/8 or .75 +.12
7	.25 + .12 or ¼ + 1/8	.25 + .12 or ¼ + 1/8	17	1	1
8	1/2 or .5	1/2 or .5	18	1	1
9	1/2 or .5	1/2 or .5	19	1	1
10	1/2 or .5	1/2 or .5	20	1 = 1/8 or 1 + .12	1 = 1/8 or 1 + .12

Parts of the aspirin 1/8 = .12, ¼ = .25, ½ = .5, ½ + ¼ = ¾ or .75, lbs. = pounds

- mg per 1/8 or .12 of a tablet = 10 mg
- mg per ¼ or .25 of a tablet = 20 mg
- mg per ½ or .5 of tablet of a tablet = 40 mg
- mg per ½ + ¼ = ¾ or .75 of a tablet = 60 mg
- mg per 1 tablet = 81 mg

For dogs in pain, give 5 mg per pound (10 mg/kg) every twelve hours. Watch for any toxicity that might develop during the aspirin administration—and stop if you cause vomiting or any other abnormality.

Or:

For anti-inflammatory, antirheumatic fever, give 11 mg per pound of body weight (25 mg/kg)—one morning and one evening. After a dog has been treated for heartworms, give aspirin at 3–4.5 mg per pound of body weight (7–10 mg/kg) by mouth once a day for not more than ten days.

Normally your veterinarian will give directions if he or she feels further treatment is necessary. If so, they will probably use better, more effective drugs.

Table 14.2 *Aspirin Dosage for Dogs*

Aspirin is not recommended for cats.
Use enteric-coated aspirin.

Caution: Due to availability of aspirin in only 81 and 325 mg tablets, it is impossible to be accurate with dosages, so dosing is ballpark because you have to cut the tablets into quarters or halves. For safety, anything under five pounds should have a prescription for pain meds from the doctor. For pain, give every twelve hours.

Weight pounds	Low Dose 4.5 mg/lbs. 81 mg tablet	High Dose 11 mg/lbs. 325 mg tablet	Weight pounds	Low Dose 4.5 mg/lbs. 325 mg tablet	High Dose 11 mg/lbs. 325 mg tablet	Weight pounds	Low Dose 4.5 mg/lbs. 325 mg tablet	High Dose 11 mg/lbs. 325 mg tablet
5	.25	.25	26	.25	1	46	.75	1+.5
6	.25	.25	27	.25	1	47	.75	1+.5
7	.25	.25	28	.25	1	48	.75	1+.5
8	.5	.25	29	.25	1	49	.75	1+.5

Weight Pounds	Low Dose 4.5 mg/lb. 325 mg tablet	High Dose 11 mg/lb. 325 mg tablet	Weight Pounds	Low Dose 4.5 mg/lb. 325 mg tablet	High Dose 11 mg/lb. 325 mg tablet	Weight Pounds	Low Dose 4.5 mg/lb. 325 mg tablet	High Dose 11 mg/lb. 325 mg tablet
9	.5	.25	30	.5	1	50	.75	1+.75
10	.5	.25	31	.5	1	51	.75	1+.75
11	.5	.5	31	.5	1	52	.75	1+.75
12	.5	.5	33	.5	1+.25	53	.75	1+.75
13	.75	.5	34	.5	1+.25	54	.75	2
14	.75	.5	35	.5	1+.25	55	.75	2
15	.75	.5	36	.5	1+.25	56	.75	2
16	.75	.5	37	.5	1+.25	57	.75	2
17	1	.5	38	.5	1+.25	58	.75	2
18	1	.5	39	.5	1+.25	59	.75	2
19	1	.75	40	.5	1+.5	60	.75	2
20	1	.75	41	.5	1+.5	61	.75	2
	Low Dose 4.5 mg/lbs. 325 mg tablet							
21	.25	.75	42	.5	1+.5	62	.75	2
22	.25	.75	43	.5	1+.5	63	1	2
23	.25	.75	44	.5	1+.5	64	1	2
24	.25	.75	45	.5	1+.5	65	1	2
Weight Pounds	**Low Dose 4.5 mg/lb. 325 mg tablet**	**High Dose 11 mg/lb. 325 mg tablet**	**Weight Pounds**	**Low Dose 4.5 mg/lb. 325 mg tablet**	**High Dose 11 mg/lb. 325 mg tablet**	**Weight Pounds**	**Low Dose 4.5 mg/lb. 325 mg tablet**	**High Dose 11 mg/lb. 325 mg tablet**
66	1	2+.25	78	1	2+.75	90	1+.25	3
67	1	2+.25	79	1	2+.75	91	1+.25	3+.25
68	1	2+.25	80	1+.25	2+.75	92	1+.25	3+.25
69	1	2+.25	81	1+.25	2+.75	93	1+.25	3+.25
70	1	2+.5	82	1+.25	2+.75	94	1+.25	3+.25
71	1	2+.5	83	1+.25	2+.75	95	1+.25	3+.25
72	1	2+.5	84	1+.25	3	96	1+.25	3+.25
73	1	2+.5	85	1+.25	3	97	1+.25	3+.25
74	1	2+.5	86	1+.25	3	98	1+.5	3+.25
75	1	2+.5	87	1+.25	3	99	1+.5	3+.25
76	1	2+.5	88	1+.25	3	100	1+.5	3+.5
77	1	2+.5	89	1+.25	3			

I WANT A FIRST-AID KIT FOR MY PETS

This is a great idea. Let's discuss some simple things to do before attempting to aid an injured pet. When working on any pet, be aware that animals will bite. They react first, and if you're in the way, you will be on the receiving end.

Some simple immunizations can make an animal go berserk. Just wiping a leg can stimulate a vicious bite—even if you own the animal. I have seen owners bitten when trying to settle pets down. It is best to let the pet settle down before sticking your hands near the pet.

Do not be sorry—just cool it and keep your hands to yourself. When it hurts, a pet will not yell, "Stop!" They bite—and the bite can be darn hard and hurt like crazy. I have a few scars to prove my point from pets that would never ever bite anyone—according to the owner. If you believe that, prepare to be bitten.

One bite I received was from a corgi. Its leg was held and wiped clean after a blood draw—and it bit me. The dog's bite was quicker than the eye, and the medical treatment cost $3,568.78. It hurt like crazy and bled a lot. Before doing the kind thing for a wounded pet, muzzle it with gauze roll. You may be glad you did—and if you do not, you may be sorry. You could also get a trip to see your physician or a visit to the emergency clinic (where the costs are much higher). The bill follows, and you will dig deep in your pocketbook. It is like a bullet—you cannot put it back once it is fired.

Your goal with first aid is to stabilize the animal so the pet can be transported for further treatment if needed. If the pet is to be transported to a veterinary facility, a simple call will alert them so they will be waiting for you.

A first-aid kit might include many things. This list is a darn good start. There may be some other items you would like to include—and by all means, do so. Most of these items can be obtained at grocery stores, Walmart, pharmacies, and many military PX and BX facilities. You might check with pet stores (Petco or PetSmart) to see if they have prepared pet first-aid kits for sale. It is easy to find a pet first-aid kit online.

Table 14.3 *First-Aid Kit Contents*

- hydrocortisone cream
- first-aid guide
- eyedropper or syringe
- gauze pads
- gauze roll or bandage roll
- hydrogen peroxide
- thermometer
- petroleum jelly
- tweezers
- iodine or betadine
- triple antibiotic ointment
- small bottle of eye wash
- insect sting pad for sting relief
- disposable rubber gloves
- tape
- small pair of scissors
- small wrapped alcohol pads
- small bottle of sterile water (but tap water will be better than nothing)
- tourniquet (or rubber tubing)
- small towel or cloth
- PetClot or QuikClot—to stop bleeding quickly
- Q-tips

OMEGA-3 OILS FOR PETS

Recent news says omega-3 fatty acids do not have the benefit on the heart muscle in people if omega-3 fish oil capsules are taken. That is popular information this month, but who knows what they will say in a month or a year. Dr. Oz (a physician on TV) says to take omega-3. I also believe there are significant benefits for dogs and cats that have nothing to do with heart or cardiac tissues.

Some supplements are pitched as a see-all, end-all. A supplement is neither one. It is a supplement, and it has some benefit. Sometimes it is not very noticeable, but it makes a big difference in the long run. Keep in mind that a supplement such as omega-3 is not a proven medical drug that is used to cure anything. It does have some effects that are of *some* benefit. We will point out some benefits for pets that have been determined by scientific studies. It must be emphasized that it is not a compound that is going to heal anything, but it seems to definitely have benefits that help some pets.

There are many sources of omega-3 oils. Capsules are available at Costco, BJ's, Walmart, grocery stores, pharmacies, and vitamin shops. We happen to feed Nordic Naturals at a dose of .75 cc on the food daily along with Hill's Science Diet to my cat. The cat's coat shines bright, and he is a very healthy cat. We also have the cat at the doctor's office every six months for a checkup and maintain a good healthy condition. I have to do what I preach.

Why do I like Nordic Naturals omega-3 for pets? It comes in convenient containers with the dosage on the side of the package and in a form that is easy to dispense. It is very simple. The company makes a special effort—like Hills Pet Food—to be among the best there is.

John Bauer, DVM, PhD, DACVN, wrote a great paper in the December 11, 2011, *Journal of the American Veterinary Medical Association* in conjunction with the American College of Veterinary Nutrition. He detailed several studies that showed the benefits of omega-3 acids, mainly docosahexanoic acid (DHA) and eicosapentanoic acid (EPA). Studies in people have shown that it reduces formations of blood clots and helps raise HDL cholesterol while dramatically lowering triglycerides.

Omega-3 can be found in lots of foods—including salmon, herring, mackerel, bluefish, and sardines—or pills. What benefits does the omega-3s have in pets? Benefits have been seen for skin inflammatory conditions such as atopy, excess fat in the blood (hyperlipidemia), heart disorders, and osteoarthritis. The benefits of the omega-3 supplements have been found to be worth the cost and effort.

Dr. Bauer's final comments on the supplementation with

omega-3 fatty acids states, "Omega-3 fatty acids as an *adjunct* to several clinical disorders have been evaluated to a greater extent in dogs than in cats." Please note that he did not say it helps—not *treats*—these conditions. There are many unknowns still to be discovered and proved or disproved, but it seems prudent to use omega-3 fatty acids.

TREATMENT

If you choose to supplement with omega-3 fatty acids—and you purchase them as people products at Costco, BJ's, grocery stores, Walmart, or pharmacies—the daily dose would be based on 180 mg for every ten pounds (180 mg per 4.54 kg) of body weight of EPA of the omega-3.

The concentration of the omega-3 is written on the bottle, and the dose of 180 mg would have to be adjusted according to the concentration of the capsules purchased. The capsules would have to be cut, and you might get closer to a dose than you think you would be giving.

The varied concentrations of purchased omega-3 fish oils makes it impossible to make a chart that is usable and accurate for all the different brands that might be purchased. Any time pills or capsules have to be split or cut, it is as close as you can come because there is no way to be accurate. One actually gets more on their fingers and hands than in the pet food.

The best option might be to drain the tablets into a container and dispense the oil from the container. Unfortunately, I have not tried this and have no idea of the difficulties this procedure might cause. The simple way is to use the Nordic Naturals.

The following dosage chart is courtesy of Nordic Naturals. They have done research to establish a daily dose with a fixed concentration of omega-3 fatty acids. The product comes with the daily dose written on the box and on the bottle with a dropper that allows the most accurate dosing possible. I use it because of the simplicity of dosing. It is done in seconds, and it is the most accurate you can be with the proper daily dose of omega-3 fatty acids. I have no connections to them or any financial gains to be had, but you will be able to dose your dog or cat simply and appropriately. Nordic Naturals can be purchased at 1-800-PetMeds (1-800-738-6337).

I have no financial gains from any source of over-the-counter products.

Table 14.4 *Omega-3 Fatty Acids Chart*

Doses in the charts are courtesy of Nordic Naturals.
Suggested daily dose for dogs
one teaspoon = 5 ml (4600 mg)

Weight	Serving	Servings per Bottle	EPA	DHA	Total Omega-3s
2–4 lbs. (.9–1.8 kg)	0.25 cc or ml	240	35 mg	21 mg	71 mg
5–9 lbs. (2.2–4.0 kg)	1.0 cc or ml	60	138 mg	83 mg	285 mg
10–19 lbs. (4.5–8.6 kg)	2.0 cc or ml	30	276 mg	166 mg	570
20–39 lbs. (9–17.6 kg)	0.5 teaspoon (2.5 cc or ml)	189	345 mg	207 mg	713 mg
40–59 (18–26.7 kg)	1.0 teaspoon (5.0 cc or ml)	94	690 mg	414 mg	1426 mg
60–79 (27.2–35.8 kg)	1.5 teaspoon (7.5 cc or ml)	63	1035 mg	621 mg	2139 mg
80–99 (36.2–44.9 kg)	2.0 teaspoon (10 cc or ml)	47	1380 mg	828 mg	2952 mg
100 lbs. (45.35 kg)	3.0 teaspoon (15 ml)	31	2070 mg	1242 mg	4278 mg

lbs. = pounds, kg = kilograms, cc = ml or ml = cc

Suggested daily dose for dogs
Use soft gel capsules for every twenty pounds (9.0 kg) of body weight.

Weight	Serving	EPA	DHA	Total Omega-3s
20 lbs.	1 soft gel	150 mg	90 mg	310 mg

Suggested daily dose for cats
one teaspoon = 5 ml (4600 mg)

Weight	Serving	Servings per Bottle	EPA	DHA	Total Omega-3s
2–4 lbs. (.90–1.8 kg)	0.25 cc or ml	249	35 mg	21 mg	71 mg
5–9 lbs. (2.26–4.0 kg)	0.5 cc or ml	120	69 mg	41 mg	143 mg
10–14 lbs. (4.53–6.35)	0.75 cc or ml	80	104 mg	62 mg	214 mg
15–20 lbs. (6.8–9.0 kg)	1.0 cc or ml	60	138 mg	83 mg	285 mg
Over 20 lbs. (9.0 kg)	1.25 cc or ml	48	173 mg	104 mg	356 mg

lbs. = pounds, kg = kilograms, cc = ml or ml = cc

TOXICITY OF IVERMECTIN

Ivermectin has been reported to poison control centers hundreds of times due to people purchasing the product without knowing how much or how long to use it. This is a major reason for writing this book and others that have been published. They provide dosages for some over-the-counter drugs for folks who will not take their pets to a veterinarian and tend to treat their own pets. It is also relevant for those who are financially strapped and need to reduce expenditures.

It is obvious that too much of a drug is harmful. It seems that some people think if a little is good, then a whole bunch should be wonderful. That "stinking thinking" leads to poisoning your pet. To aid in preventing this from happening, Table 14.5 provides proper dosages of Ivermectin for dogs and cats. All one has to know is the weight of the pet—and then look up the dose in cc. Give only the dose recommended in cc for the weight of the pet—and no more. *Do not overdose—it kills pets.*

Ivermectin can be used to treat red mange (demodex skin

infections), prevent heartworms, treat heartworms and many internal parasites, such as hookworms, roundworms, and whipworms. It is important that proper dosages be used or you can kill your pet or make your pet very ill. Causing death or illness is unnecessary; just follow the dosages provided within the pages of this book. Collie breeds are much more sensitive to Ivermectin than cats and other dogs are.

If you have read *How to Treat Your Dogs and Cats with Over-the-Counter Drugs Companion Edition,* you have read that not all collie dogs have the gene for sensitivity to Ivermectin. You can have your dog tested by mail at the College of Veterinary Medicine at Washington State. The veterinary college has a simple mail-in test. The book describes in detail all you need to know to get your dog tested for the gene if you desire to do so.

Follow dosage recommendations—and do not overuse drugs in your pets!

TREATMENT
Dosage charts for Ivermectin can be found in Table 14.5 for ear mites, scabies, heartworm, hookworms, roundworms, whipworms, and lice. Look up the pet's weight and obtain the dose in cc from within the chart. Remember not to overdose. Only give the dose that is on the chart.

For demodex, different dosages are used. See the three different dosage charts below (Tables 14.6, 14.7 and 14.8) for day-one demodex, day-two demodex, and the dosage chart for demodex for days 3–14 and longer if needed.

PREVENTION
Prevention of overdosing with Ivermectin is easy if you use the dose in cc indicated for the weight of your pet on the Ivermectin charts.

Table 14.5 1 Percent Ivermectin Dose-by-Weight Chart

(weight divided by 80 = dose in cc)
Use for heartworm prevention and for *nondemodex*
skin mites, roundworms, hookworms, whipworms,
and threadworms (Strongyloides).
Do not overdose!

Weight Pounds	Dose cc	Weight Pounds	Dose cc	Weight Pounds	Dose cc	Weight Pounds	Dose cc	Weight Pounds	Dose cc
1	0.01	21	0.26	41	0.51	61	0.76	81	1.01
2	0.02	22	0.27	42	0.52	62	0.77	82	1.02
3	0.03	23	0.28	43	0.53	63	0.78	83	1.03
4	0.05	24	0.30	44	0.55	64	0.80	84	1.05
5	0.06	25	0.31	45	0.56	65	0.81	85	1.06
6	0.07	26	0.32	46	0.57	66	0.82	86	1.07
7	0.08	27	0.33	47	0.58	67	0.83	87	1.08
8	0.10	28	0.35	48	0.60	68	0.85	88	1.10
9	0.11	29	0.36	49	0.61	69	0.86	89	1.11
10	0.12	30	0.37	50	0.62	70	0.87	90	1.12
11	0.13	31	0.38	51	0.63	71	0.88	91	1.13
12	0.15	32	0.40	52	0.65	72	0.90	92	1.15
13	0.16	33	0.41	53	0.66	73	0.91	93	1.16
14	0.17	34	0.42	54	0.67	74	0.92	94	1.17
15	0.18	35	0.43	55	0.68	75	0.93	95	1.18
16	0.20	36	0.45	56	0.70	76	0.95	96	1.20
17	0.21	37	0.46	57	0.71	77	0.96	97	1.21
18	0.22	38	0.47	58	0.72	78	0.97	98	1.22
19	0.23	39	0.49	59	0.73	79	0.98	99	1.23
20	0.25	40	0.50	60	0.75	80	1.00	100	1.25

Table 14.6 Day-1 Demodex Dose-by-Weight Chart

1 Percent Ivermectin Dosing Chart
(weight divided by 100 = dose in cc)

Weight Pounds	Dose cc	Weight Pounds	Dose cc	Weight Pounds	Dose cc	Weight Pounds	Dose cc	Weight Pounds	Dose cc
1	0.01	21	0.21	41	0.41	61	0.61	81	0.81
2	0.02	22	0.22	42	0.42	62	0.62	82	0.82
3	0.03	23	0.23	43	0.43	63	0.63	83	0.83
4	0.04	24	0.24	44	0.44	64	0.64	84	0.84
5	0.05	25	0.25	45	0.45	65	0.65	85	0.85
6	0.06	26	0.26	46	0.46	66	0.66	86	0.86
7	0.07	27	0.27	47	0.47	67	0.67	87	0.87
8	0.08	28	0.28	48	0.48	68	0.68	88	0.88
9	0.09	29	0.29	49	0.49	69	0.69	89	0.89
10	0.10	30	0.30	50	0.50	70	0.70	90	0.90
11	0.11	31	0.31	51	0.51	71	0.71	91	0.91
12	0.12	32	0.32	52	0.52	72	0.72	92	0.92
13	0.13	33	0.33	53	0.53	73	0.73	93	0.93
14	0.14	34	0.34	54	0.54	74	0.74	94	0.94
15	0.15	35	0.35	55	0.55	75	0.75	95	0.95
16	0.16	36	0.36	56	0.56	76	0.76	96	0.96
17	0.17	37	0.37	57	0.57	77	0.77	97	0.97
18	0.18	38	0.38	58	0.58	78	0.78	98	0.98
19	0.19	39	0.39	59	0.59	79	0.79	99	0.99
20	0.20	40	0.40	60	0.60	80	0.80	100	1.00

Table 14.7 Day-2 Demodex Dose-by-Weight Chart

1 Percent Ivermectin Dosing Chart
(2 times per day, 1 dose = dose in cc)

Weight Pounds	Dose cc	Weight Pounds	Dose cc	Weight Pounds	Dose cc	Weight Pounds	Dose cc	Weight Pounds	Dose cc
1	0.02	21	0.42	41	0.82	61	1.22	81	1.62
2	0.04	22	0.44	42	0.84	62	1.24	82	1.64
3	0.06	23	0.46	43	0.86	63	1.26	83	1.66
4	0.08	24	0.48	44	0.88	64	1.28	84	1.68
5	0.10	25	0.50	45	0.90	65	1.30	85	1.70
6	0.12	26	0.52	46	0.92	66	1.32	86	1.72
7	0.14	27	0.54	47	0.94	67	1.34	87	1.74
8	0.16	28	0.56	48	0.96	68	1.36	88	1.76
9	0.18	29	0.58	49	0.98	69	1.38	89	1.78
10	0.20	30	0.60	50	1.00	70	1.40	90	1.80
11	0.22	31	0.62	51	1.02	71	1.42	91	1.82
12	0.24	32	0.64	52	1.04	72	1.44	92	1.84
13	0.26	33	0.66	53	1.06	73	1.46	93	1.86
14	0.28	34	0.68	54	1.08	74	1.48	94	1.88
15	0.30	35	0.70	55	1.10	75	1.50	95	1.90
16	0.32	36	0.72	56	1.12	76	1.52	96	1.92
17	0.34	37	0.74	57	1.14	77	1.54	97	1.94
18	0.36	38	0.76	58	1.16	78	1.56	98	1.96
19	0.38	39	0.78	59	1.18	79	1.58	99	1.98
20	0.40	40	0.80	60	1.20	80	1.60	100	2.00

Table 14.8 Days 3-14 (Maybe More) Demodex Dose-by-Weight Chart

1 Percent Ivermectin Dosing Chart
(day-1 dose times 3 = dose in cc)

Weight Pounds	Dose cc	Weight Pounds	Dose cc	Weight Pounds	Dose cc	Weight Pounds	Dose cc	Weight Pounds	Dose cc
1	0.03	21	0.63	41	1.23	61	1.83	81	2.43
2	0.06	22	0.66	42	1.26	62	1.86	82	2.46
3	0.09	23	0.69	43	1.29	63	1.89	83	2.49
4	0.12	24	0.72	44	1.32	64	1.92	84	2.52
5	0.15	25	0.75	45	1.35	65	1.95	85	2.55
6	0.18	26	0.78	46	1.38	66	1.98	86	2.58
7	0.21	27	0.81	47	1.41	67	2.01	87	2.61
8	0.24	28	0.84	48	1.44	68	2.04	88	2.64
9	0.27	29	0.87	49	1.47	69	2.07	89	2.67
10	0.30	30	0.90	50	1.50	70	2.10	90	2.70
11	0.33	31	0.93	51	1.53	71	2.13	91	2.73
12	0.36	32	0.96	52	1.56	72	2.16	92	2.76
13	0.39	33	0.99	53	1.59	73	2.19	93	2.79
14	0.42	34	1.02	54	1.62	74	2.22	94	2.82
15	0.45	35	1.05	55	1.65	75	2.25	95	2.85
16	0.48	36	1.08	56	1.68	76	2.28	96	2.88
17	0.51	37	1.11	57	1.71	77	2.31	97	2.91
18	0.54	38	1.14	58	1.74	78	2.34	98	2.94
19	0.57	39	1.17	59	1.77	79	2.37	99	2.97
20	0.60	40	1.20	60	1.80	80	2.40	100	3.00

USE AND DISPOSAL OF MEDICATIONS

Everyone has had medication dispensed to them for a pet. The problem is that the directions that come with the prescription are not followed. The medication dispensed is for the purpose of helping the pet. The biggest issue with medication is that it is stopped before all of it has been used according to the directions on the label. The most common reason is that the pet has stopped showing signs of the condition for which the medication was dispensed.

What is the big deal with stopping when the signs are no longer present? When medication is used, it takes a few days for the medication to start to have an effect. The pet will start to feel better in a few days as the medication starts to have its magical effects. That is because the medication has "beaten up" the cause of the disease, and the signs have diminished. The lack of signs does not mean that the cause of the disease has been eliminated. Not completely wiping out the cause of the disease produces resistant bacteria and other resistant organisms. Use medications—as directed—until the end.

It goes without saying that medications need to be properly stored—out of the way of children and pets. Some pets open medications and eat it all at once. This happens with pet medications and people medications. Just a few days ago, we had a client whose dog opened a childproof container and consumed all the medication in the bottle. She was mad that she had to pay for a refill. It happened because she did not keep her medications away from her pets. Do not share medications. Each patient has different conditions, needs for certain medications, and specific dosages.

When the pet is well, it is time to dispose of medications that have not been used for some reason. It should not be flushed down the toilet. There are a lot of folks disposing of medication every day. Medications cannot be easily removed from water, and the medications build up in the environment. Different areas have different rules for disposing of medication. A call to the county or municipality that controls waste can inform you how they want you to dispose of medicines.

TREATMENT

Medication is for the treatment of a condition in your pet, and it is important that the directions on the prescription are followed correctly.

PREVENTION

Safe storage of medications—away from children and pets—is very important.

PRECAUTIONS WITH MEDICATIONS

Medication overdosing is a problem for owners treating their own pets. Thousands of pets are reported to poison centers ever year because they have been unintentionally poisoned. The goal of this and other books is to help reduce the numbers of poisoned pets by providing information that good-intentioned owners can use to treat their pets safely.

Without good, appropriate information, a person has no clue about what drug to use, how much medication to give, or how many days to use the medication. The result is a dead pet or a very ill pet. The pet could have survived, but it was poisoned.

One of the goals of this book is to help folks with limited knowledge about the use of over-the-counter drugs and their appropriate dosage to enable them to use the drugs correctly. This book has the necessary information to allow pet owners to use over-the-counter drugs safely. Within these pages, you find descriptions of diseases or conditions that are aimed at providing you with the necessary information to allow you to proceed with the proper treatment (not every treatment possible) safely and effectively.

Pets become a part the family, and they are our buddies. We want the best for them. It is important that you approach the issue with the idea that you will do the best you can for your pet. The best alternative for the treatment of your pet is the pet's doctor. Veterinarians have been extensively trained in the art of veterinary medicine for the sole purpose of animals. A veterinarian is always the best approach for medical information and treatment.

When using any drug, it is important that the proper diagnosis is made so that one knows what is to be treated—and that the correct drug for the condition is used. Understanding the condition that you intend to treat is essential. The next step is deciding on the medication that is to be used for the condition you have decided needs your treatment.

After the selection of medication is made, the proper amount of the drug must be determined. This is one of the most important steps—and your full attention can prevent you from overdosing your pet. Drug dosing is based on an amount of drug per pound or kilogram of the pet. It takes a bit of math to calculate the proper dosage. In this book, this step has been done for you. All you need know for the proper dosage is the weight of your pet. Look up the pet's weight. Only give your pet the correct dosage. *Do not overdose your pet.*

TREATMENT

Treat every pet according to the treatment dose by weight that is presented in this book. Do not overdose your pet since the pet's health is of paramount importance.

PREVENTION

I believe it is best to have a good preventive medicine program since there is no way to see the future. Early diagnosis of any condition is the best one can do for a pet. I realize that there are some people who feel that they cannot afford such a service, but I know that prevention is much cheaper than treatment. Treating your pet yourself is an option that requires proper knowledge and proper use of over-the-counter drugs. However you do it, we hope for the very best for your pet.

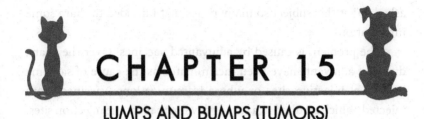

CHAPTER 15

LUMPS AND BUMPS (TUMORS)

In real life, I assure you there is no such thing as algebra.
—Fran Lebowitz

All tissues in the body have cells that die, and new cells take their place. The process goes on and on. Sometimes there are little bumps or small traumas that occur, which may not even be noticeable because they are internal. When this happens, the body starts to mend itself. A part of mending is the production of more blood vessels at the point of trauma to expedite the healing.

When the wound has healed, the extra blood vessels that came to the aid of the wound normally go away. However there are times when the blood vessels hang on. Those blood vessels continue to provide nutrition for tissues and stimulate the growth of new cells. These new cells are almost always abnormal. Not all cancer gets a start this way, but several do. The new growth could be malignant or benign—and it may go away with time or continue to grow.

Most new cells continue to grow, and more blood vessels develop to feed the new growth. In this chapter, we will discuss different lumps and bumps that occur in pets. We will identify the stimulus for the tumor or abnormal tissue growth and discuss some growths that are spread by contact. We will also cover different varieties of cancers that occur in pets.

INJECTION-SITE (ISS) OR VACCINE-ASSOCIATED SARCOMA (VAS)

I had no intention of writing about this subject, but I have been asked about this subject so many times that I decided to share some information.

The problem is caused by adjuvanted vaccines. Over the years, different adjuvants have been incriminated as the cause of sarcoma tumors at injection sites or where immunizations (vaccines) were injected, which resulted in a tumor development at the injection sites. The terms used for this syndrome are either Injection-Site Sarcoma (ISS) or Vaccine-Associated Sarcoma (VAS). The different terms are minor in the big picture, but VAS seems to be more commonly used.

A vaccine contains an adjuvant, which is the cause of the tumor development and not the disease-preventing part of the vaccine. The disease-prevention portion of the vaccine is non–tumor producing. Tumors develop at the injection site. Early tumor development appears as a small inflammatory reaction. When you see this inflammatory reaction, it should be removed. I would not wait. Later seems to be too late for successful treatment. My opinion is just that—an opinion—not a scientific fact.

The major problem has been in immunized cats that were given rabies vaccines or Feline Leukemia Vaccines (FeLV). Both vaccines have been the cause of several tumors. Rabies immunizations have caused the largest number of tumors (most likely due to the fact that a rabies vaccination is required by law in many states). It is the owner's decision to vaccinate for FeLV.

These two vaccines account for the majority of tumors produced by vaccination. However, any adjuvanted vaccine can cause tumors, even though it may have a low incidence of occurrence. I have immunized thousands of pets and have never seen one tumor. This does not mean it does not happen. Perhaps this clinical observation reflects a low incidence of tumor occurrence. Furthermore, there is some thought and agreement that adjuvant vaccine injection-site tumor development may have a genetic basis for causing susceptibility to vaccine-associated sarcoma development. If your pet develops a sarcoma at the injection site, it is a very disappointing, frustrating, and expensive experience for you and your pet.

Antibodies are the soldiers that protect against disease organisms. The antibody fixes bayonets and kills the invading disease agents—be it virus or bacteria. In the case of the disease we are discussing, it kills or eliminates the virus and prevents the diseases.

What is an adjuvant? An adjuvant is an agent that enhances antibody production (antigenicity) of a disease-preventing particle. An example is the extra stimulation of a portion of a virus or bacteria to cause more protection of stronger and greater numbers of antibodies. To prevent illness, these extra antibodies are able to close with and destroy the disease-causing organisms. The adjuvant is not the disease-preventing part of the immunization. The disease virus or part of the virus in the vaccine is the antibody producer. The adjuvant makes the virus or part of the virus a better antibody producer.

If you had high-school chemistry or college chemistry, you might remember that a "catalyst" makes a reaction work better or faster but is not involved in the reaction. Adjuvant makes the immunization stronger by allowing more antibodies to be made, but the adjuvant is not an antibody producer. By itself, it would not produce any antibodies, but it is the causative agent that causes cancer.

TREATMENT

Treatment is by surgically removing the mass or tumor; if it is caught early, the chances are better for treatment. This is an invasive and spreading type cancer. As it spreads or metastasizes, the cancer causes large masses in the lungs. It is an ugly disease. Once tumors get started, reoccurrence is high (ranging from 30–70 percent).

PREVENTION

The best prevention is not to allow any adjuvanted vaccines to be given to your pets. There are vaccines that do not have adjuvants in them. Injection-site or vaccine-associated sarcoma incidence may be low, but it is very significant if it happens to your pet. Early recognition of a skin issue at any injection site should prompt you to see professional help quickly.

MAMMARY TUMORS

Mammary tumors account for about 70 percent of all tumors in dogs and can be benign or malignant. Some breeds of dogs are somewhat more prone to mammary tumors than others are. Those more prone to tumors—spaniel breeds, English setters, Maltese, Yorkshire terriers, pointers, dachshunds, Doberman breeds, and German shepherds— seem to be more prone to malignant mammary tumors. There may be some genetic causes involved in mammary tumor development.

If a dog is spayed before the dog has a heat cycle (estrus), tumor incidences are low (in the neighborhood of only 0.5 percent). If the dog has one cycle and is spayed, the incidence of mammary tumors is about 8 percent; if it is done before two years of age, the incidence is about 26 percent. Therefore, from a tumor point of view, it is advisable to have a female dog spayed before the first heat cycle. For those with male dogs, the incidence in males is less than 1 percent.

Advancing age increases tumor occurrence in nonspayed dogs. The median age of incidence of mammary tumors is plus or minus seven to eleven years of age. However, for malignant tumors, the incidence is roughly around 9.5 years compared to nonmalignant tumors at around 8.5 years of age.

The good news is that if you have your female dog spayed before a heat cycle, you significantly decrease the possibility of mammary tumors. Of course, there are no guarantees, but the data is on your side.

If you notice a lump on or by the mammary glands, my surgery experience tells me that it is time to remove it. The sooner the animal is spayed or neutered, the better. What seems like a simple small lump probably already involves the entire chain of mammary tissues. If you are lucky, it may only be local. My surgical experience with mammary tumors has shown that if there is a mammary lump, there is much more involvement in the mammary tissue than you can see on the surface.

Some people say, "Wait until it grows." If you're concerned about the health of your pet, this approach is a bunch of baloney. You need to have any growth removed yesterday. The bad news is that waiting may allow deep invasion by the tumor into adjacent tissues—or it may spread to other parts of the body. You do not want to wait—just do it!

TREATMENT

This condition requires your pet's doctor for help in dealing with mammary tumor growths. As stated above, I believe your pet should have surgery as soon as you can schedule it to have *any lumps removed*—the sooner, the better. My opinion is due to my surgical experiences with mammary tumors.

If financially possible, follow-up chemo treatment may be needed and helpful. Under any circumstance, surgical removal of any growth in the mammary gland region is advised. We all hope you never have to deal with these kinds of issues.

PREVENTION

The best prevention is having your pet spayed at an early age—and at least before two years of age. If at all possible before the first heat is the best you can do. Hormones (progesterone and estrogen) play an important part in tumor development. Progesterone and estrogen influence greater than 90 percent of benign tumors. Early spaying helps prevent mammary tumors.

LUMPS UNDER THE SKIN (LIPOMA)

Frequently, a lump develops under the skin that seems to stop growing after reaching a certain size. However, there can be others that seem to become quite large. Many are of concern to owners since they appear as tumor growths—and owners should be concerned. There is no way to tell what a lump of growth under the skin is by just looking at it. Lumps may appear anywhere on the body with no special reason for having occurred. The mass feels soft—and perhaps fluid.

Whenever there is a growth under the skin, it is a good idea to have it checked out by the pet's doctor. It can be a simple benign mass on the body or a pocket of serum called a seroma. Frequently, it can be a growth of fat that is benign (lipoma). A lipoma normally will not be an issue for a pet. However, some lipomas seem to just keep getting larger. Most remain small, but others grow quite large. The largest I operated on was a little larger than a softball or the size of a large man's fist. Why owners wait that long is a mystery to me. The dog had two of them—one on the front of the chest and one on the right side of the chest.

Most lipomas occur in middle-aged and older dogs, and it is rare in cats. Overweight dogs may be more prone to developing lipomas, and female dogs may be more prone to lipoma development under the skin. If a lipoma appears in a cat, it is more likely to occur in a male cat.

The mass is normally small and solitary, but there can be multiple masses. Most usually feel soft and frequently feel like squeezing a small liquid cyst. A lipoma may cause compression of adjacent organs when it occurs within the abdomen or thorax. Those that develop within the thorax or abdomen have no signs to let one know that the growth is present—and they can completely fill the abdomen or thorax.

I have done thousands of abdominal surgeries and have found only one dog with internal lipoma that completely filled the abdomen. The fat was not greasy and was rather firm. Frequently these growths under the skin seem to be ignored by owners and may have been present for a year or more before calling the pet's doctor.

Diagnosis is very easy. With a needle aspiration, the doctor squirts the tissues onto a microscope slide so the fat can be observed. If it happens to be a seroma, the fluid is removed—and the mass is gone—but it can reoccur. It may take three or four aspirations of a seroma for it to stop coming back.

TREATMENT

The treatment for a lipoma is surgical removal, which normally does not grow back. It can do so if it is not all removed. Normally the removal is the end of the lipoma. Unlike mammary tumors, the lipoma is not an expanding tumor under the skin. It is almost always local;

if stable, it may not need surgery. However, to be safe, it is better to have a good diagnosis of the mass and have it removed if necessary. Be sure—not sorry; a malignant tumor may look and feel like a lipoma.

PREVENTION

Since a lipoma is a spontaneous growth—and the trigger for growth is not known—there is little an owner can do to prevent it. Overweight dogs are more prone to lipoma; losing excess weight is always good for the health of the pet.

TRANSMISSIBLE VENEREAL TUMOR OF DOGS

Transmissible tumors of dogs can be very common in the dog population if dogs are left to run outdoors without supervision. The disease is spread by sexual contact with animals that have the transmissible venereal tumor within their genitalia.

The tumors often bleed and can protrude from male or female genitalia. The tumor is cauliflower-like in appearance. The tumors are benign and normally do not spread. If they do spread, normally it is just to the regional lymph nodes. The tumors often become very large and extensive within the genitalia. The tumors are almost always located within the animal's genitalia.

The tumors may be deep inside the genitalia; when an animal is examined, it can be overlooked due to the small size and location deep in the prepuce or the vagina.

The tumor is transplanted from site to site and dog to dog by direct contact. Metastasis is rare, but it has been noted in kidneys, spleens, eyes, brains, pituitary glands, skin, below the skin (subcutis), intestinal lymph nodes, and in the abdominal lining (peritoneum).

TREATMENT

Spontaneous regression can occur, but it takes a long time—if it happens at all. Most often, the tumor is treated by surgical removal, radiation therapy, and chemotherapy. Total remission normally occurs with a minimum of six treatments. Surgery alone is not effective since there are small areas that cannot be accessed for surgical removal—and it will regrow.

PREVENTION

Prevention is the best option and can be achieved if one supervises the dog when it is outside to prevent dog-to-dog contact.

ULCERS ON THE UPPER LIP OF CATS

Ulcers on the upper lip of cats seem to be quiet common; they are often referred to as rodent ulcers. The name rodent ulcer dates way back to a time when it was believed that cats obtained these ulcers by catching rodents, mainly rats and mice.

Today, they are called *eosinophilic ulcers*. These ulcers are normally located on the upper lip above the canine teeth or longest tooth in the upper mouth. These can be found over one tooth, or both sides can be involved. The ulcers can be small or large, causing the upper lip to bulge out. The ulcer can be seen easily. The size is relative to the length of time the ulcer has been present.

The most common cause of rodent ulcers is an allergy. Common allergens that cause ulcers are insects, fleas, or food. Other types of contact allergies have been considered imitating agents. In all probability, the most common cause is flea allergy due to a lack of treatment. There are reports indicating that the allergy causing the ulcers may be inherited. Since there are so many different locations that develop different eosinophilic-type lesions, it is believed that different tissues may be more prone to different types of ulcers. Since the ulcers are open wounds, they can become infected due to secondary infectious bacterial invaders.

Eosinophils are a type of circulating blood cell. Rodent ulcers have an increased number of eosinophilic cells present in the lip ulcers.

TREATMENT

This is an issue for your pet's doctor to tackle. Treatment can be frustrating. However, persistence and patience will save the day. It is stated that this ulcer will go away without treatment. I have never seen this regression or healing without the aid of treatment. Along with treatment, a good flea program should be initiated with monthly treatment for fleas.

PREVENTION

A good flea-treatment program will do wonders for avoiding rodent ulcers. This is another condition that would be picked up early with a good wellness plan and most likely would never occur. Since this may be an inherited condition, cats with rodent ulcers should not be bred.

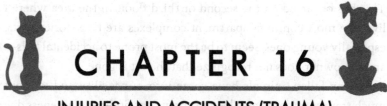

CHAPTER 16

INJURIES AND ACCIDENTS (TRAUMA)

Whether you think that you can, or that you can't, you are usually right.
—Henry Ford

Injuries are things that often could be prevented with simple supervision of pets outdoors or in areas that may invite trauma. A big trauma producer is an accident between a pet and a moving vehicle. We see broken legs, broken backs, smashed pelvises, eye popped out of heads, broken ribs, skin de-gloved, and many other traumatic issues—and all could have been avoided if the pet had been on a leash and had supervision.

Another common injury is putting a collar on a pet and letting the pet grow without looking at the collar again. The collar becomes embedded in the skin and can be up to six inches deep; it is sad but true. Some people put rubber bands, string, or wire on a pet and forget about them. The poor pet is cut by the tight foreign body and grows with the foreign body embedded in the skin.

Not treating for ear mites results in the poor cat or dog mutilating its neck or ears from scratching. In this chapter, we will discuss traumatic events and their aftermath for the poor pet who suffers the consequences of mistreatment or neglect.

THROWN OR FALLING PETS FROM
HIGH-RISE APARTMENTS

I have seen dogs that have been thrown from high-rise apartments. This has occurred on the second or third floor. In the area where I live, the most common apartment complexes are two stories. Cats, especially young ones, seem to be the most prone to accidental falls—and the owner does not recognize that the cat is gone.

Many fallen animals have come into our facility and without much trauma or damage. The most prevalent finding is lameness due to broken bones and some minor bleeding from the mouth, which may not even be present the next day. The unfortunate ones may have broken bones and lung issues. This might include open wounds in the lung tissues. The diaphragm, which separates the lungs from the intestines, may be ruptured. The intestines can be in the area of the lungs with associated abdominal hernias. In high-rise apartments, it would seem that those that fall from higher floors would have more traumas—but not nearly as much as one would expect.

Those that are thrown have a forward and then a down motion in the fall; and the most common pet to experience this are young dogs. They sometimes survive fairly well from two stories, but obviously the higher the plunge, the more traumas. When examining a fallen pet, expectations are to find all kinds of serious issues, but frequently it is not really so bad (considering that the poor pet has just experienced a rather traumatic fall). It is not advisable for owners to throw their pets anywhere.

Many falling pets are due to leaving doors or windows open when a pet is in the apartment or two-story home and the owner is not paying attention to the pet. An analogous issue in our area is when parents with pools are not paying attention to young children—and terrible things happen. Pets falling from two stories and higher causes too much trauma in the pet for survival, and death rates run about 90 percent in all animals that fall or are thrown from these heights.

Cats falling from six or seven stories can hit sixty miles per hour, which creates one whale of an impact. Some cats have rather surprisingly low trauma issues, but others die on collision. This is most likely due to the way the body hits the ground—and perhaps how rigid or relaxed the pet is at impact. The good news is that if a fallen cat can make it through the first two days, it has a better than average chance of surviving.

TREATMENT

Never throw pets out doors or windows—and certainly not from upper floors of apartment buildings. Most of the cats that fall are young, but it does occur with older cats as well. Fallen pets are the result of open windows or doors and neglect. Keep doors and windows closed to keep the pet from dangerous areas, which are most often out the back of the building. Patios can be screened in, which makes a nice outdoor area for cats.

The cat that falls could be yours—so be alert and take precautions to make sure it is not your pet that falls. I know a person who was cat sitting on a second-story window with a screen on it—and the cat *still fell*. It accidentally pushed out the screen and landed on top of her van!

Screens are not always able to secure cats. If you have screens, you need to make sure they are secured so cats cannot pry the screens open. This little trick may save you a lot of heartache.

PREVENTION

Folks who have thrown their pets out doors or windows at higher elevations are often reacting to a pet doing something, which makes the owner angry. Take a deep breath, count to ten, and remember that whatever mess the pet made will have to be cleaned up if the pet is thrown out or not. Just do not throw a pet. Keep possible escape areas, such as windows and doors to the outside, closed when supervision cannot be given—and it just will not happen. A fallen pet is normally a dead or traumatized pet.

INJURED FOOTPADS

The footpads are of a special kind of skin that is tough compared to normal skin of the animal. This allows the animal to walk on many different kinds of surfaces with ease and without pain.

This discussion will focus on what can be done if there is an injury or complete removal of this special footpad tissue. Injury to footpads can include cuts, bruises, thorns, foreign bodies, or even complete traumatic removal of footpad tissues. There may be other causes. The bottom line is that trauma to the feet of pets often results in painful lameness that needs attention.

The type of injury will normally dictate the necessary treatment. A cut may need a triple antibiotic ointment and a bandage. Bruises can be a cause of lameness; depending on severity, treatment may only require limited activity or cage rest until the pet overcomes the lameness caused by the bruise.

A hunting dog that may not have been outside much can run its footpads off, and a pet in a traumatic incident can have the footpads torn off. There are many ways that footpads may be traumatically removed from one or more digits of the foot. The removal of a footpad will not only cause pain—it will produce lameness in the foot involved. The first treatment is to clean the wounds, apply a triple antibiotic ointment to the wounded footpads, and bandage the foot.

There are animals that will remove the bandage faster than you can put it on. If this is what you experience, an Elizabethan collar may keep the pet from chewing at the bandage. If you can keep the pet somewhat confined, you will have done about all you can do.

There are finger splints available at pharmacies, CVS, Walgreens, and Walmart. They can be found in grocery stores or even dollar stores. If you can find one that will cover the pet's foot, give it a try by bandaging the finger splint over the wound on the dog's foot. The finger splints tend to be aluminum. It makes the bandage harder to get off. However, animals that remove bandages are experts at removing them quickly.

Normally, in just a few days, there will be improvement—or at least less lameness will be noted. There is a product that can be used to toughen the footpad tissues. Tuf-Foot is available online at www.tuffoot.com Tuf-Foot is a liquid and is easy to apply. Use a cloth or small amount of cotton and moisten with Tuf-Foot and apply to the footpads. This will burn on freshly traumatized tissues, and the pet will react to the application since it burns when applied to raw fresh tissues.

If you know you will be taking a pet to an area that might cause trauma to footpads, you can plan ahead. You can apply Tuf-Foot ahead of time to toughen up the footpads. Tougher footpads help prevent traumatic events from occurring.

Tuf-Foot is a brown liquid; if you apply this to your pet's feet in your home, you might have dog tracks across your carpet or furniture.

TREATMENT

Treatment is dictated by the kind of injury that is present; start with ointments and bandaging. Following triple antibiotic ointment, treat the footpads with applications of Tuf-Foot. The Tuf-Foot will toughen the footpads. Applying Tuf-Foot to raw tissues will burn, and your pet will react quickly to the pain if you do this. Remember that any bandage on a foot or leg may be too tight, and you can cut the circulation and cause more trauma. After an hour or so, check to see if the foot or leg is swelling. If so, redo the bandage—but do not make it so tight.

PREVENTION

It is always best to have good supervision whenever your pet is outside. If going hunting, prepare by applying Tuf-Foot ahead of time to toughen up the feet. Tougher footpads mean less trauma to the feet of the pet. Tuf-Foot is available at www.tuffoot.com.

SNAKEBITES

The bad news is that being bitten by any snake is not good. Poisonous and nonpoisonous snakes will bite—and both can be infectious. Poisonous snakes cause the most trauma to the victims. At times, it may be difficult to determine if the bite is poisonous or nonpoisonous.

In some areas of the United States, bull snakes closely resemble prairie rattlesnakes and can make the same noise as a rattlesnake. A bull snake has infectious materials in its mouth that are transferred to a bitten animal. The nonpoisonous bite often requires antibiotics for treatment of local infections, and careful observation is necessary to make sure it was not a poisonous bite.

There are numerous species of pit vipers and coral snakes, and the numerous names of different snakes and taxonomy will not be a subject of this discussion.

The most common snakebites are from rattlesnakes, copperheads, and cottonmouth snakes. All are known as pit vipers. In different areas in North America, these snakes can be different sizes. The amount of venom injected into a victim depends on the size of the snake, time since its last bite, and duration of the bite.

I have treated many snakebites, and there is seldom bleeding at the site of the wound—unless it happens to penetrate a blood vessel. The locations of the fang marks have never been hard to find, but hair and color of the pet makes finding the fang marks a bit difficult. The bites of pit vipers normally come with swelling that occurs very quickly.

As a side note, I remember a case being referred to UC Davis Veterinary Hospital. It was actually a rat poison consumption case. This case points out the fact that there can be confusion upon deciding upon the cause of the problem. The poisonous bites of pit vipers rapidly cause swelling, pain, and discoloration of the skin. Depending on the location, the swelling may cause difficulty breathing (due to tissue swelling).

Most often, the owner is not present when the pet is bitten—and there is no knowledge of the type of snake that has bitten the pet. Cats are worse than dogs since cats tend to hide after being bitten. Cats may get bitten once and go back for another look and get bitten more than once. If the snake is very quick, it might strike twice. I have never seen a cat that was bitten more than twice. Those bitten twice have very poor prognosis, but they can survive. The sooner the bite is treated, the better.

Another danger in the snake world in North America is the coral snake. There is a saying used to identify coral snakes: *Red and black is friend of Jack; red and yellow kill a fellow.* This refers to the colors that are touching each other. This snake, like the king cobra, has a neurotoxin that affects the nervous system and causes relaxation of muscles. The response in the medical world is known as a curare effect. It is just like the darts used in the jungles by natives for hunting with blow darts. These snakes are shy and seldom are involved in a bite, but it happens. Some pets when picked up will have the snake attached—and still biting. The snake bites with a chewing action. The bite is not nearly as painful as a pit viper bite, but it is deadly.

The most common signs of coral snakebites that may be noticed by an owner are difficulty breathing, paralysis of the limbs, or collapsing. The pet becomes flaccid, just like with tick paralysis, botulism, or coonhound paralysis. The other signs are subtle and require a professional to recognize them since many are not very noticeable and may require tests.

Death is normally due to failure of respiration due to the muscle paralysis. The good news is that about 60 percent of coral snakebites do not inject venom. You have no way of knowing this—so do not hesitate. If you know your pet was bitten, act quickly; later may be too late to save the pet.

With any condition, early recognition of a problem is necessary to enable treatment; the quicker the treatment is started, the better the chance the pet has of pulling through.

TREATMENT

As with many health conditions, the treatment for a coral snakebite will vary. The nature of the snakebite will require the expertise of the pet's doctor to enable a chance of survival from the snake's venom. The vaccine for rattlesnake bites will not cover all species of rattlesnakes but does protect for most. The vaccine may be available at your pet's doctor's clinic. The American Animal Hospital Association recommends that dogs less than sixteen weeks of age receive two immunizations a month apart. Dogs over sixteen weeks of age should also receive two immunizations a month apart. The immunization requires an annual booster.

PREVENTION

Not allowing a pet to roam without supervision in areas that may have poisonous snakes is the best one can do. Hunters who let dogs go may put their pets at the most risk. The good news is that fewer dogs are bitten.

In some areas, bites are extremely common. I once treated more than fifty pets with pit viper bites in less than twelve weeks.

FIRE ANTS

Fire ants bite dogs and cats. The bites produce skin lesions from multiple stings, which a single ant can inflict on the skin of a pet. After the first fire ant sting, it rotates sideways and stings again. The ant repeats this process several times and will have attached itself with the mouth parts and sting six or seven times in a circular motion.

The stinging motion of the ant creates a painful lesion. The sting damages the skin (necrosis) and has an allergen associated with the venom within the sting. The allergen can react with pets that happen to be allergic. The allergic pet has an even greater reaction to the venom than other animals might experience. All of this damage may come from one ant, and the problems are multiplied by the many ants that might get on the pet.

Reactions can cause local infected lesions (pustules) and even anaphylaxis and death of the pet. A red or erythematous lesion forms quickly after the stings have been completed. One can tell how recently the bites have occurred by the appearance of the lesions. The skin becomes red in about one minute. In about two hours, the lesion becomes moist (papule); within four hours, the skin is raised due to small blister-like formations. Fluid accumulation (vesicles) occurs at the sting site. As the blisters are forming, the fluid inside the blister is clear, but by eight hours, it is cloudy.

At about twenty-four hours, the blisters will become infected and be filled with pus (exudate) due to infection. There is almost immediate pain produced by the stings of the ants, which cause a very itchy feeling. The pet may start biting and scratching at the area. This phenomenon often becomes less intense in about an hour. However, during the time that the pet experiences the itching sensation, the skin can become damaged from the biting and scratching, making infections of the skin even worse. More severe reactions will require a trip to the pet's doctor for proper care and treatment.

TREATMENT

Ice or compresses of cool water or rubbing alcohol can be of some help in reducing pain. Ointments with combinations of different compounds—such as antihistamines, triple antibiotics, and ointment—that have pain relievers, such as lidocaine or other topical pain reducers, have been effective in helping treat the bite wounds. In uncomplicated cases of fire ant attacks, most pets do well with these types of treatments. If the treatments are not working and the lesions get worse, it is important to seek help from the pet's doctor before serious problems happen.

PREVENTION

If you live in an area with fire ants, the best prevention is to ensure that your pet does not have the opportunity to meet up with them. If you have fire ants in your lawn, consider service companies that can treat the yard; this will normally eliminate the ants from your yard for a full year. Remember that some pets can have serious reactions to fire ants and will need to see the doctor quickly if the pet is to be saved.

CHAPTER 17

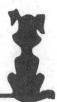

SOMETHING OLD, SOMETHING NEW, SOMETHING BORROWED, AND SOMETHING BLUE

Three may keep a secret, if two of them are dead.
—Benjamin Franklin

Some things do not fit under a specific subject heading but will be found in this chapter. It is a hodgepodge collection of some facts and different subjects thought to be of interest to pet owners. Ever wonder why cat hair seems softer than dog hair? Why does it take a long time for hair to grow back in? This chapter also includes a summary of all the drugs discussed in this book. There are some other goodies to go with it.

MY CAT'S LITTER BOX

A few years ago, pets were not allowed in homes. Almost all pets were outside pets or indoor-outdoor pets. Times have changed, and many animals are kept indoors almost all the time. In fact, many people now purchase clothes for their pets. When immunizing cats or dogs, owners often ask if the clothes should be removed; this normally is not necessary.

The indoor cat creates issues for normal animal waste. For cats, it is often a litter box that is made available for a bathroom. The type of litter is not important—as long as the pet will use the litter provided by the owner. Some cats will not use scented litters. If not, try another until the cat is satisfied with the product you provide. When trying out different litters, purchase small amounts to determine the type your cat will actually use. If you are not successful, try another brand of litter. Some cats will be good in the litter, and others are sloppy—but at least it is used.

The next issue is keeping the litter clean. The cat may stop using the litter, and excrement may be found around the house. If this happens, it may lead to a learned behavior, which may be very difficult to correct. Another cause of not using a litter box is a urinary infection. Many cats will squat—and nothing happens. This is normally due to a bladder infection.

Clients frequently say, "I think my cat is constipated; she tries, but nothing happens."

The cat's doctor can diagnosis this problem and prescribe the necessary medicine. Do not hesitate since this can become a serious problem if left untreated.

Cleaning the litter is rather easy. The owner should accumulate the necessary tools to keep the litter fit for use. Tools for maintaining litter are available at many stores, such as Walmart, Petco, PetSmart, and other retail stores. There are electric litter boxes that clean fifteen minutes after the cat uses the litter box; it dumps wastes into a plastic container with a lid that closes for easy disposal. Automation is simple and the easiest way to keep litter clean. If one cleans the litter manually, it should be done daily.

A special note to pregnant women: Cat litter should not be handled during pregnancy due to the potential for toxoplasmosis infection of the fetus. Use the automatic litter box for family health reasons, ease of cleaning, and maintaining sanitation within the household. If you do not have an automated system, it may be a great birthday or Christmas gift in the near future.

Automated cat litter cleaning systems can only handle a limited number of cats. A large population of cats is more than one system can handle. Manual systems might be a better way to go in a multiple-cat household.

TREATMENT

Keep the litter box clean. A urinary tract infection can also be a cause of not using a litter box. This will require medication that can be provided by the pet's doctor. Get the pet looked at to rule out urinary infections.

Male cats can have a blocked urethra that prevents urination. A blocked urethra has been the cause of death for dogs within two days. Do not hesitate—just do it!

WHAT TO EXPECT FROM A WELLNESS PLAN

This description of a wellness program is my opinion; every veterinary practice will have some deviations from the following programs. However, if the program offered does not meet with your expectations, you are within your rights to dictate to your veterinarian what you want accomplished with your wellness program.

A pet wellness plan is for the sole benefit of your pet's health; normally such a program will involve several procedures. The first for any wellness program is the all-important blood work, including a complete blood count (CBC) and blood chemistry. A complete physical exam at each visit is necessary—regardless of the age of the pet.

Dogs and cats age faster than people do—and their organs deteriorate at a much faster rate than people's do. A CBC is a part of the baseline of healthiness for pets and is a must to keep on top of your pet's health. A CBC will detect infections, anemia, and platelet numbers. It will detect some bleeding disorders and help determine dehydration. It also detects any malformed red cells, which are the oxygen-carrying cells, as well as other conditions.

Blood chemistry reveals the conditions of the liver, kidneys, electrolytes, the correct balance between sodium and potassium, and blood calcium levels, and it detects pancreatic issues if present. Depending on the type of blood machines the veterinary practice has, there may be more or less test results recorded. The blood work provides an important baseline and organ function information about your pet.

Many disease processes do not happen all at once. The disease condition can be developing slowly; without health checkups, there is no way to determine that a condition is developing. With blood work on file at your pet's doctor's office, a slowly developing health condition can be detected and corrective actions can be started to prevent the condition from developing into a severe health condition. The doctor can simply compare previous blood data with the most recent results. Unfortunately, without frequent health checkups, this type of diagnosis is not even possible.

Depending on the age of your pet, the following chart includes basic guidelines. It is broken down into young, middle age, and old. I choose to let your veterinarian decide what is young, middle age, and old since there are always differences of opinions.

Table 17.1 *Suggested Physical Exam Parameters by Age*

Young	Physical exam, CBC and blood chemistry panel, fecal exam
Middle Age	Physical exam, CBC, blood chemistry panel and urinalysis, fecal exam
Senior	Physical exam, CBC, blood chemistry panel, urinalysis, thyroid testing, blood pressure, electrocardiogram, and fecal exam

There are several benefits to a wellness program for your pet:

- A wellness program establishes healthy baseline values.
    - o Many cats and dogs will show subtle changes in blood values over time.
    - o Blood value changes cannot be detected without the benefit of previous blood tests.
    - o It is important to have the baseline at a young age so values can be compared as the pet ages.
- A wellness program can identify an unseen disease at an early stage.
    - o Finding a disease before clinical signs appear increases the

>   chances for success in preventing further development of the conditions.
>   o   Finding a disease early can lessen the cost of treatment.
>   o   Early identification of a health issue prevents waiting for obvious signs to develop.
> • A wellness program serves as a preanesthetic health screen for any surgery or dental procedures.
> • A wellness program is beneficial to patients receiving or starting medication.
>   o   Blood work on file helps avoid administrating medications that might be unsafe for the pet.
>   o   Regular blood tests will help identify unwanted side effects that can occur with some medications.

IN MY TIME

The art and science of veterinary medicine has improved and advanced exceptionally in the short years since I graduated from veterinary college. We have moved from glass syringes to plastic disposable syringes—and from needles that had to be sharpened to disposable needles that are very sharp. There are obvious reasons for these improvements in the profession of veterinary medicine, and it seems that all areas have advanced.

Veterinary colleges have had monumental advances in their educational and professional training programs. New students are graduating with the best education in the history of the profession. A new graduate has impressive, in-depth knowledge when he or she leaves the halls of learning. This medical training and knowledge is a solid foundation that sets the stage for the profession of veterinary medicine.

Continuing education organizations have kept pace and have even advance the pace of providing education. Each year, they help thousands of doctors update their knowledge, learn new techniques, and stay abreast of the equipment changes for use in diagnosing and treating animals in the modern age. The continuing education meetings are very impressive and have very large selections of subject matter to present to all kinds of specialties and general practice veterinary doctors.

In my time, there have been advancements in research for improved medications and new knowledge of diseases that were not even known or taught when I graduated. These events have been phenomenal. Some diseases were left untreated due to lack of medications; demodex skin mites come to mind quickly. I remember many poor animals that were so badly infected and looked awful due to lack of medications available. Modern medicines have changed this significantly, thank goodness, and it is far better for the animals. Medications have been the tip of the iceberg for advancement in the profession.

I believe the major change has been board specialties. This phenomenon has brought on excitement and mountains of new information along with advanced expertise in many disciplines. Board specialization covers surgery, dermatology, ophthalmology, neurology, and emergency medicine—and there are many more. In each of the board specialties, there are subspecialties, such as a surgeon specializing in bone or soft tissue surgery or a veterinary ophthalmologist specializing in cataracts or posterior eye problems. All this is due to the concentration on these special areas requiring more and more knowledge to be able to make a difference for those animals in need of this type of medical treatment. This new need has resulted in improved knowledge and techniques never before imagined.

I find that people do not understand the expansion in veterinary expertise and knowledge, and they are surprised to learn of board specialties in veterinary medicine. I believe it has proven to be an essential need for the advancement of knowledge and expertise in modern veterinary medicine. In the modern age of robots, unmanned vehicles, and mountains of information on medical issues, it is impossible to be a know-it-all. This is due to the extensive in-depth knowledge and expertise that now exists. It is a very exciting time in veterinary medicine. This does not mean that there is no need for general practice doctors—there is a huge need. It is my belief that general practice veterinary medicine will eventually be a board specialty.

There are areas that lag because of remoteness and low-practice income limitations, such as isolated areas where tumbleweeds are four miles apart, which need large-animal services. More and more programs are being initiated to provide these areas with large-animal veterinary services.

Sir Winston Churchill said, "Now this is not end. It is not even the beginning of the end. But it is, perhaps, the end of the beginning."

DEFINITIONS

SIGNS VERSUS SYMPTOMS

It is time for a couple definitions or clarification. By definition, animals cannot have symptoms. Animals have "clinical signs" that are often referred to as signs. A symptom can be described by a person, but an animal cannot describe the pain or the location of any issue. However, if an animal's foot hurts, it may limp as a sign of a problem of the leg, foot, or toes.

To be correct when referring to animal issues, we need to refer to signs instead of symptoms. In actuality, the words are often used incorrectly to refer to the same thing. The dictionary definition of symptom is "any indication of disease perceived by the patient" and is therefore not applicable to animals. The expression used instead is "clinical signs"

RADIOGRAPH VERSUS X-RAY

We often call the image of an x-ray procedure an x-ray. In reality, the image on film or computer is a radiograph that was produced by x-rays as they penetrated the body and caused an image to occur. This image is correctly called a radiograph. An x-ray is a particle that is generated and expelled from an x-ray machine.

An x-ray is a high-energy electromagnetic radiation produced by the collision of a beam of electrons with a metal target in an x-ray tube. A radiograph is a film produced by radiography.

WHY CAT'S HAIR IS SOFTER

The computer has much information about dog and cat hair. I am astounded by all the ambiguousness and nonsense found online. This useless pontification does fill a purpose; it clogs the information highway with junk. It is something to read and immediately disregard about dog and cat hair. I read one entry that stated there are three kinds of hair: long hair, short hair, and no hair. *Oh my,* I thought, *if she had called Geico, she could have saved some money.*

There are three kinds of growing hairs:

1. Anagen hairs are new hairs.
2. Catagen hairs are middle-aged hairs.
3. Telogen hairs are the older hairs that have stopped growing and are waiting to be replaced by younger hairs.

Hair does not all grow at the same rate—and certainly all do not grow at the same time. Old grandpa-type telogen hairs are constantly being replaced with new anagen hairs. This is the cycle of life for hair.

Each animal has what are known as guard hairs and secondary hairs. Guard hairs are seen on dogs and are primarily telogen hairs. Cats have primary secondary hairs that are primarily anagen hairs (new hairs). The secondary hairs give cats the soft, velvet-like feeling when compared to dogs.

CUT SLOW-GROWING HAIR

Have you ever seen or had a dog that had its hair cut—and it seems never to regrow. Why is this? Most of the visible hair on a dog is telogen hairs. When cut, they are ready to be replaced. Hairs grow slowly, and do not all grow at once. A clipped area may have patches that come in here and there before it is all replaced. It can take up to about three years for some dogs to replace the cut hair.

SPINES ON THE MALE CAT'S PENIS

Spines on the penis of a male cat will appear at about twelve weeks of age. The spines cover the glands of the penis; the point is directed toward the back of the cat. Penile spines will be absent from cats that are neutered (castrated) at about six weeks after surgery. The spines are dependent upon testosterone for development and spine persistence.

DIAGNOSING FLEAS THE EASY WAY

An easy way to diagnose fleas is to put a 3x5 white card behind and next to the tail head. Scratch dander and debris onto the card, and a little black speck may be seen on the card. Wet your hand and let a few drops of water drop onto the card—and you may see red streaks from the little black dots. The little black dots are flea feces, which is dried blood. The drops of water that drip from your hand dissolve the black specks of dry blood, and you will see streaks of red blood. When you see the red streaks, you have your diagnosis of fleas. This is not a 100 percent sure way, but it is often a very fast, effective way to diagnose fleas

THE BEST WAY TO GET BACK A LOST PET

The best way to get back a lost pet is to have your pet chipped—and get it registered. You can register the chip by calling 1-866-699-3463. If the chip is not registered, it is just a gizmo under the skin of your pet. Be happy and get your pet back by registering your pet's chip now. If you need more help, the American Animal Hospital Association has a website you can use to look up information based on a chip number: http://www.petmicrochiplookup.org.

THE MOST FREQUENTLY REPORTED PET POISON

The leading cause of poisoning in pets has been human medications. This item has always been on top-ten lists of poisons for pets. People need to keep personal medications away from pets. Remember that what might work for your health might kill your pet. Be safe—not sad. Keep medications away from children and pets.

April showers bring May flowers, and the bunny brings Easter lilies that kill pets due to renal failure if eaten.

Table 17.2 *Summary of Drugs*

Do not overdose!
Dose, when to give, and repeat if indicated, and where to purchase.
Do not overdose; follow directions carefully.

Drug	Use	Dosage	Number of Days	When to Repeat Dose	Where to Purchase
Panacur Fenbendazole	Intestinal parasites	See dosage charts on page 218 if purchased at 100 mg/cc at feed store. If purchased elsewhere, follow directions on label.	Once daily for 3 days	In 2 weeks, repeat same dose for 3 days; if possible, repeat the fecal exam to be sure all parasites are gone	PetSmart, Petco, 1 (800)-PetMeds, feed stores, and online
1 Percent Ivermectin	Hookworms roundworms, whipworms, tapeworms, and Strongyloides	See dose-by-weight chart on page 43	1 day	Repeat in 2 weeks	Feed stores

Drug	Use	Dosage	Number of Days	When to Repeat Dose	Where to Purchase
1 Percent Ivermectin	Heartworm prevention	See dose-by-weight chart on page 43	Once monthly	Give every month	Feed stores
1 Percent Ivermectin	Demodex skin mites	See dose-by-weight charts on pages 93 day 1 – page 94 day 2 – page 95 day 3-14 and more if needed	Minimum of 14 days	Until skin scrape is negative	Feed stores
1 Percent Ivermectin	Ticks, lice, scabies, ear mites	See dose-by-weight chart on page 43	1 time for ear mites a .3 cc in each ear and massage will be of benefit	Repeat weekly for 3 weeks	Feed stores
Advantage II	Fleas	Color coded by weight of pet	Once monthly	Give every month	PetSmart, Petco, 1 (800)-PetMeds
Advantix II	Fleas, mosquitoes ticks, flies, and lice	Color coded by weight of pet	Once monthly	Give every month	PetSmart, Petco, 1 (800)-PetMeds, Online
Cat Aspirin	Cat pain and fever	See cat dose-by-weight chart on page 30	Once	Repeat in 3 days if necessary	Grocery stores and pharmacies
Dog Aspirin	Dog pain and fever	See dog dose-by-weight chart on pages 28 and 29	Morning and evening	Repeat only as needed	Grocery stores and pharmacies

Drug	Use	Dosage	Number of Days	When to Repeat Dose	Where to Purchase
3 Percent Hydrogen peroxide in dogs	Induce vomiting	½ cc per pound or 1 cc/kg	Once	If no vomiting, repeat in 5 or 10 minutes double dose 1 cc/lbs. or 2 cc/kg. Do not exceed 1.5 cc/lbs. or 5 ml/kg	Grocery stores, pharmacies, Walmart
Omega-3 fatty acids	Seborrhea	See dose-by-weight chart on page 256 dogs – 257 cats	Once daily	Most likely for life of the pet	Vitamin shops 1 (800) PetMeds Nordic Naturals 800-622-2544 x103
12.5 Percent Sulmet Sulfadimethoxine 125 mg	Coccidia	See dose-by-weight chart on page 57 day 1 – page 58 days 2-5	Day 1 dose is double day 2–5 dose	Day 2–5 are ½ the dose of day 1	Feed stores (Sulmet is in a large bottle that is also used for chickens) PetSmart, Petco, and 1 (800)PetMeds
Activated Charcoal (260 mg capsules)	Flatulence (intestinal gas)	Small dog 1–2 capsules, medium dog 1–7 capsules, and large dogs 1–12 capsule in any one day	Adjust to minimum dose that controls intestinal gas	Repeat only if indicated	Walgreens Pharmacy

ABOUT THE AUTHOR

Dr. Robert Ridgway graduated From Kansas State University College of Veterinary Medicine and completed a residency in internal medicine at the University of California–Davis. After graduating from veterinary college, he worked for a short period of time at a veterinary hospital in Topeka, Kansas. He entered the US Army Veterinary Corps where he became director of the Animal Medicine Division on Okinawa. He later completed a residency of comparative medicine at the Madigan Army Medical Center. He is a graduate of Officer Candidate School at Fort Sill, Oklahoma, and a graduate of the US Army Command and General Staff College. He was the treasurer of the District of Columbia Academy of Veterinary Medicine for fourteen years. He served as secretary-treasurer and president of the District of Columbia Veterinary Medical Association. He was the first US Army officer to be in charge of the Department of Defense Military Dog Veterinary Service at Lackland Air Force Base in San Antonio, Texas. He completed a master's of international management at the University of Maryland, University College. After retiring from the army, he worked at Covance Laboratories, Banfield Pet Hospital, and Orange County Animal Services in Orlando, Florida. Dr. Ridgway is a diplomate in the American College of Veterinary Preventive Medicine and a diplomate in the American College of Laboratory Animal Medicine. Dr. Ridgway is married and has one daughter and one male cat.

INDEX

all-meat diets, 47, 126–127, 184–185, 239

alopecia (hair loss), 14–15

amaryllis, as toxic, 178t

American Animal Hospital Association, 283, 295

American College of Veterinary Nutrition, 254

American Heartworm Society, 42

American Veterinary Medical Association, 132

American Veterinary Medical Association Journal (AVMAJ), 126, 147

amputation, as treatment for biting of body parts, 157

anagen (new hairs), 4

anal prolapse, 216–217

anaphylaxis, 71–72, 115, 284

Ancylostoma canium worm, 86t

Ancylostoma tubaeforme worm, 86t

anemia, 47, 53–54, 99, 103, 104, 117, 289

anesthesia, risks from, 213

Angels' Eyes, 10

animal behaviorists, 146

animal trainers, 146, 147, 152

animal training on your own, 147

anorexia, 39, 142, 211

ant bites, 115

anterior chamber hyphema (blood in eye), 228–229

antibiotic ointments. *See also* triple antibiotics ointments
  as treatment for hot spots, 16
  as treatment for injuries to footpads, 280
  as treatment for insect stings, 115
  as treatment for minor skin wounds, 163, 167

antibiotic-resistant bugs, 2

antibiotics
  defined, 245

impact of prolonged use of, 2
  as treatment for badly infected mouth or ulcers, 243–244
  as treatment for bubonic plague, 39
  as treatment for ear fly bites, 109
  as treatment for ear infections, 44
  as treatment for fire ant stings, 285
  as treatment for infections between toes, 18
  as treatment for Lyme disease, 65
  as treatment for Malassezia, 21
  as treatment for mastitis, 71
  as treatment for nasal discharge, 69
  as treatment for nonpoisonous snakebites, 282
  as treatment for urinary tract infection, 34

antibodies (IgE), 12

antifungal medications, 20, 21

antigen tests, 84

anus, infections around (perianal fistula), 220

arthritis, 26, 46, 166, 168, 225

artificial tears ointment, 154, 230, 231

aspirin
  for cats, 297t
  caution in using, 27
  for dogs, 297t
  dosage charts for cats, 30t, 249t
  dosage charts for dogs, 28t–29t, 250, 250t–251t
  enteric-coated, 28
  overdosing on, 246–247
  for pets, 247
  recommended dosages, 247–248
  as treatment for elevated temperature, 27

Association for Pet Obesity Prevention, 125

ataxia (unsure footing), 164, 175

atopic dermatitis (AD), 12

frequent urination, 34–35

fungal infections, of toes and toenails, 19

FUO (fever of unknown origin), 26

FURminator, 3–4, 5

FVRCP (feline viral rhinotracheitis, calicivirus, panleukopenia) vaccination, as core vaccine, 78t

G

garlic, as poisonous to pets, 182t

gas passing, 137–138

Gas X (smethicone), as treatment for flatulence, 137

generalized hair loss, 14

generalized seizures, 165

genetics, role of in development, 183–184

GenTel Gel, as treatment for dry eyes, 230–231

gentian violet, 45

gestation period, 197

giardia, 100

giardia vaccination, as not recommended, 77, 78

glucosamine, 45–47

gram diet scales, 200

granulomas, lick, 35

grape juice, as toxic, 176t

grape seed extract, as toxic, 176t

grapes, as toxic, 50, 176t, 182t

grass awns, 18, 49

Greenies (treats), 142

grooming, 3–4, 139

growth and development, 183–195

Gump, Forrest (fictional character), 213

gums

dark red, as signs of impending heatstroke, 68

pale, as sign of anaphylaxis, 72

pale, as sign of immunization reaction, 75

gunpowder, as toxic, 49

H

hair, slow-growing, 294–295

hair bristles, 18

hair loss, 4–6, 14–15, 17, 91–92

hair stain caused by eye discharge, 9–11

hairballs, 134–135, 138, 139

hairs, infected, 18

halitosis (bad breath), 135–136

HARD (heartworm-associated respiratory disease), 41

hard bones, cautions with, 238

hard chew toys, cautions with, 238

hard foods, impact on teeth of, 136, 238, 239

HBC (hit by car), 223

HDL cholesterol, 254

head tilt, 63–64

head turn, 64

heart conditions, 64, 65

heartworm prevention, 47, 82–84, 100, 191. See also Ivermectin

heartworm test, 49, 215

heartworm-associated respiratory disease (HARD), 41

heartworms, 38–39, 40–42, 47, 49, 192, 250, 258

heatstroke, 67–69

Hemingway, Ernest, 187

Hemingway cats, 187

hemobartonellosis, 53

hepatitis vaccination, as core vaccine, 77t

hernias, 217, 218–219

heterochromia iridum, 189–190

hip dysplasia, 223

Hirschsprung's disease (congenital megacolon), 189

Ivermectin
dosage charts, 43t, 85t, 93t–95t, 108t, 259t–262t
overview of, 296t–297t
as prevention for ear infections, 45
as prevention for heartworms, 42, 49, 55
toxicity of, 257–258
as treatment for demodex, 91, 92
as treatment for demodex ear mites, 111
as treatment for heartworms, 83–84
as treatment for hookworms, roundworms, and whipworms, 118
as treatment for maggots, 107
as treatment for threadworms, 120

J

joint issues, 65, 223–225
Journal of the American Veterinary Medical Association (JAVMA), 254
jumping up on people, 146

K

Kansas State University, 235
Kennedy, John F., 161
keratoconjunctivitis sicca (KCS), 230–231
kidney disease, 64
kittens
at four weeks of age, 200–204
newborns, 198–199
normal standards for, 201t
preventive medicine program for, 191–192
Klinefelter syndrome, 188
kneecap luxation, 225
K-Y jelly, 25

L

lameness, 4, 18, 64–65, 162, 166–168, 186, 224, 225, 278, 280
lead poisoning, 178t
leaving pets alone outside, cautions with, 51, 157, 167, 171
leptospirosis vaccination, as noncore vaccine, 77
lesions, infected (pustules), 284
lick dermatitis, 35–37
lick granulomas, 35
lidocaine, for treatment of bite wounds, 285
lip infections, 20–21
lipoma (lumps under the skin), 271–273
litter boxes
cautions for people cleaning, 99, 288
dirty litter box, as cause of permanently urinating outside box, 155
importance of keeping clean, 287–289
liver flukes, 100
lockjaw, 48
loose stools, persistent, 59–60
lost pet, finding, 157–159, 295–296
low-fiber diet, as treatment for flatulence, 137
low-viscosity eye medications, 231
lubricant products, 25
lumps under the skin (lipoma), 271–273
lung infections, 69
Luv My Pet (immunization clinic), 84
Lyme disease, 48, 49, 64–66
lymph node infections, 39
lymph node swelling, 65

M

macadamia nuts, as toxic, 178*t*, 182*t*
maggots, 107
malabsorption syndromes, 60
maldigestion syndrome, 60
mammary gland infection (mastitis),
  70–71
mammary tumors, 270–271
marking territory, 155–156
matting, 4–6
Maugham, W. Somerset, 123
medications
  activated charcoal capsules,
    137–138, 298*t*
  Advantage II. *See* Advantage II
  Advantix II. *See* Advantix II
  Albon (Sulfadimethoxine), 55, 104
  aspirin. *See* aspirin
  Benadryl (diphenhydramine
    HCL). *See* Benadryl
    (diphenhydramine HCL)
  benzoyl peroxide, 91
  eye medications, 231, 233
  flea medications, 100, 203*t*
  Gas X (smethicone), 137
  GenTel Gel, 230–231
  hydrogen peroxide. *See* hydrogen
    peroxide
  Ivermectin. *See* Ivermectin
  limitations of over-the-counter
    drugs, 245
  omega-3 fatty acids. *See* omega-3
    oils / omega-3 fatty acids
  oral antifungal drugs, 20
  Panacur (Fenbendazole). *See*
    Panacur (Fenbendazole)
  Praziquantel, as treatment for
    tapeworms, 118
  Praziquantel with Pyrantel
    Pamoate (Drontal or Droncit),
    as treatment for tapeworms,
    118

precautions with, 264–265
  Revolution, 55, 100, 103, 118
  storage of, 245
  Sulmet (Sulfadimethoxine). *See*
    Sulmet (Sulfadimethoxine)
  Terramycin ophthalmic
    ointment, 233
  use and disposal of, 263–264
megacolon, 189
megaesophagus (oversized
  esophagus), 139, 140
Merck Manual, 120
methicillin-resistant *Staphylococcus
  aureus* (MRSA), 2–3
methylxanthines, 175
microchipping, 158–159, 295
milk
  pasteurization, 48
  as poisonous to pets, 182*t*
mineral oil, 11
mistletoe, as toxic, 178*t*
mites
  demodex ear mites, 110–111
  demodex mites, 15, 19, 91–92
  ear mites, 64
  rabbit ear mites, 92
mitten cats, 187
mosquitoes
  as carriers of heartworms, 42,
    47, 82
  stings, 114
mothballs, as toxic, 178*t*
moving, impact of on pets, 50–51
MRSA (methicillin-resistant
  Staphylococcus aureus), 2–3
MRSP (*Streptococci pseudintermedius*),
  2
multifocal hair loss, 14, 15
mushrooms, as toxic, 177*t*

NOTES

The next twenty-five pages with lines are for you to record:
- your physical exams
- trips to the veterinarian
- breeding dates and newborns
- immunizations and dates (and by whom)
- other information as you see fit
- recorded veterinary costs
- dates and types of surgery

Suggested physical checklist:
- head
- eyes—eyelids, clearness of the eyes, third eyelids (if not visible, leave it alone)
- ears
- mouth, teeth, gums, throat, tongue
- neck
- chest
- back
- legs
- feet
- tail
- hair/coat
- anus
- genitalia